PRAISE FOR
Why I Hated Pink

In her first publication, Maryellen Brisbois, a brilliant nursing leader and educator, finds herself with the diagnosis of breast cancer. This is not just another breast cancer survivor story, in journal format; she very candidly shares with us her breast cancer story from diagnosis, treatment, and recovery. It is a private journey told with dignity and a respectful recount of family thoughts, medical decisions, and discussions.

Lisa C. Strazzullo Riha, Family & Community Health

Nurse Brisbois boils down her cancer diagnosis at age 41 into one-page (and less) bites in her candid, wry, and encouraging memoir. Her life with *The Fucker* (the name her sister first called the tumor) will strike reminiscent chords with those who have been there. As Brisbois states, "If I do the best I can every day, there is nothing else I can ask of myself."

Bette-Lee Fox, Library Journal

Telling a life: Recommended Reading
A nurse and nursing instructor suddenly ends up being a breast cancer patient (who knows way too much).

Mark Rotella, Publishers Weekly

In her compelling story of survival, Maryellen shares the intimate details from each point of her journey back to health from initial diagnosis through chemo treatments, from waiting rooms to hospital theaters, from family reactions to day-to-day struggles, all written with refreshing honesty and warmth.

Maryann Yin, Galley Cat

Anyone whose life has been touched by cancer will appreciate Maryellen's wit. She battles cancer with the rare insight of a person who understands that life is too absurd to take seriously and too precious to waste. She laughs far more often than she cries and never loses sight of what's important in life ~ her three children, her husband, her vast network of family and friends, and being able to laugh at yourself no matter how bad it gets.

Shelly Aucoin, Vitality Magazine

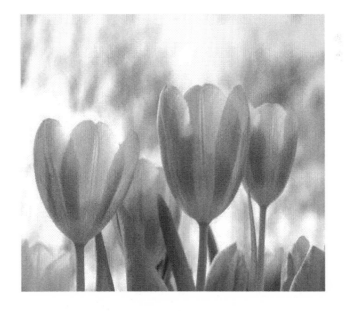

Twelve Octobers

Reflections of a Breast Cancer Survivor

• MARYELLEN D. BRISBOIS •

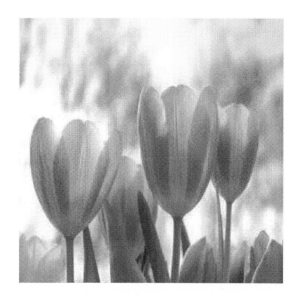

ISBN-13: 978-1547214679
ISBN-10: 1547214678

"Women agonize over cancer;

we take as a personal threat the lump in every friend's

breast."

- MARTHA WEINMAN LEAR
  Permission to publish the quote has been requested

· author's note ·

The names and other identifying characteristics of some of the person's included in this memoir have been changed.

· kudos ·

The writing of part two of this story would not have been possible had it not been for the expert care I received, the overwhelming love and support of family, friends, and strangers, and for my desire to keep the 'cloud' of cancer at bay, while holding fast to my last shred of dignity.

I am forever indebted to, and in awe of, men and women who have a recurrence of cancer as soon as they get their sea legs under them. I am acutely aware that without an overabundance of luck and damn good health insurance, I could have been or might be in a similar situation one day and will follow their daring lead.

Along the way, I have met the most extraordinary people who have become connected due to circumstance. We have laughed and cried, doing our best to get through. These 'pinkies' have inspired me to be better and do better. I have silently but deeply mourned the loss of many, as I would a dearest friend; without ever having met in person.

To my 'daughters,' 'sisters,' soulmates, aunts, cousins, grandmothers, great grandmothers, mother in law, and especially my beautiful mom Eleanore, who always encourage me to be myself. Thank you all for the love.

And to my 'sons,' 'brothers,' friends, uncles, cousins, father in law, and husband Brian who make everything right. And finally, to my dad Paul, who I know is always near and slaying dragons from afar.

I am the luckiest woman in the world.

- Maryellen D. Brisbois

• foreword •

The foreword to 'Twelve Octobers' was written by my son Tyler for an assignment in his Freshman Writing class in college.

STUFFED SHELLS

Jimmy Stewart and Charlie Brown

I have been compared to my grandfather since the day I was born. I inherited his thick dark hair and am told that I had a similar hairstyle to that of Ernie from Sesame Street the day I was born. I guess it's a stretch of a compliment at best. Our thin frame and George Bailey-like persona have always been looked upon as identical. I can thank my mother for these traits, whom is a spitting image of my grandfather. Proof of genetics. Like brown hair, cancer has to do with genetics. Unlike brown hair, cancer is far from a desirable characteristic. It's like a family heirloom that no one wants.

My most vivid memory of my grandfather was when I was three. My brother Travis and I were playing with a small building set on my grandparents' living room floor. I broke one of my brother's pieces, and all I can remember is my grandfather's disappointed voice. He wasn't angry, nor did he raise his voice. He was disappointed which is far worse than anger. When I think about it, I can't recall what he said but I can see him sitting in his recliner perfectly. In my mind, his words are muffled by time and sound like the teacher from the *Peanuts*, frustrated "whah, whahs." Unfortunately, it's the only memory of him that I have.

Years later, I remember rummaging through my closet and, for whatever reason, discovered the broken piece that was the only one from the entire set that had survived many years of spring cleaning.

Regrettably the unpleasant has a tendency of sticking around with us. Why couldn't the unbroken pieces make it? They weren't busted. Why couldn't I have a more meaningful memory of my grandfather? Even in the short three years I knew him, I know there were countless of them. He passed away after a five-year battle with leukemia.

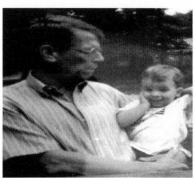

Grandpa and Me 1994 (Photo courtesy of my Mom)

Yesterday
There is always an event every few decades that defines a generation, a landmark number on the calendar that connects the masses. The baby boomers are identified with the John F. Kennedy assassination in 1963; my generation with September 11th. Anyone that was older than three for either of those dates could tell you where they were, whom they were with, and will always begin or end their story with the cliché, "I remember it like it was yesterday."

But it's true; I could tell you everything about that day. I was in Mrs. Fitzpatrick's fourth grade class on a Tuesday when I found out about the attacks on New York City and Pennsylvania. I guess the mind has a way of capturing all these little details on the days we would prefer to forget. In eighteen years, I've only had one other of these unofficial "yesterdays."

Stuffed Shells
I still remember sitting at the kitchen table (my Mom recalls
me standing) as the words *breast cancer* fell from my mother's
sentences. I remember cringing almost as if snow had fallen
down my back. The foul word was then followed by a gentle
bombardment of more filthy words such as chemotherapy and
radiation. The next eight months of our family's life was laid
out in front of me like a blueprint; an agenda from hell.

During my mother's treatment, she wrote small stories that
were later compiled into a memoir of her experiences. One of
her first short stories she explained how she broke the news to
my brother and me. She told of how strong I was and how
well I took the news, a fourteen-year-old in shining armor if
you will. I'm glad I will be forever romanticized in a piece of
literature because I can tell you that this is far from the truth.
The word tears never made it to my page of glory.

Maybe her version is right and maybe I am wrong (all I know
for sure is that we had stuffed shells that night for dinner). But
I can't be, I remember it like it was yesterday.

Holding on Tight
Everyone has had that horrendous combination of fear and
uncertainty at one time or another. Sitting at that table I've
never experienced the feeling so strong. The only feeling I can
compare it to would be like riding one of those rickety
wooden roller coasters at one of the carnivals that stay in town
for a week at most. Oh, and you just ate syrupy cotton candy
and overpriced popcorn right before you've mustered up the
courage to pull that rusty bar down over your lap. There's
nothing you can do but go along for the ride. Every single
drop puts your stomach up past your heart. But even this
doesn't compare to how I felt the next several months.

Just a Day at the Beach
The other day in my Microbiology class we learned that the word cancer originated from *Karakinos*, the Greek word for crab. Hippocrates noticed that the inside of tumors looked similar to the outline of the crustacean. I couldn't see the resemblance, but I couldn't think of a better thing to name the disease after. It comes out of nowhere and bites you on the ass while you're enjoying a beautiful day at the beach, enjoying life. That's what cancer did to us: bit us right on the ass.

Hating Pink
My mother's diagnosis came only a few months after my best friend's Mom passed away from breast cancer. I can remember looking at his empty desk, as I realized why he wasn't in school. I prayed I was wrong, but in the back of my mind, I knew I wasn't. She had three sons, one my brother's age, one my age, and one my sister's age. She had battled cancer for as long as I could remember. During her treatments, members of the community would help by making dinners. And I'm not sure why, but I remember my mother making their family stuffed shells.

When something is on your mind it seems to appear all over the place, in places that you had never noticed them before; a terrible game of hide-and-seek. Those little pink ribbons were in magazine articles, newspaper advertisements, canned goods at the supermarket, shampoo commercials, etc. And every single company seemed to be donating to breast cancer causes around the time of my mother's diagnosis. It's like they all jumped on the bandwagon once it happened. Of course, they had always been there, you've looked at them, but never took the time to see them. There was no escaping cancer. No escaping the pink. My mother's memoir is called *Why I Hated Pink*, properly named if you ask me.

Torn Pair of Genes
My mother's cancer had nothing to do with genetics.
Actually, it had nothing to do with anything. Besides my
grandfather, there was no family history or any outstanding
risk factors that made her more prone than anyone else.
"Just bad luck," the doctor had said. I guess that's one way to
put it.

Card Tricks
Doctors base a cancer patient's survival rate on a five-year
increment. They give a percentage of the chance that the
patient will live for the next five years. When I think about this
systematic benchmark, all I can picture is a bunch of doctors
sitting in a poorly lit room with short, smoldering cigarettes in
their mouths at a poker table flipping over cards, handing out
these unwelcomed numbers to terrified patients. A Hollywood
hybrid between 'The Sting' and television show 'Scrubs.' I
don't know what my mother's 'magic number' was, but I
know for a fact it wasn't one hundred percent and that scares
the hell out of me.

I don't know if it was a blessing or a disadvantage that my
mother had been a nurse for over twenty years when she was
diagnosed. I guess in a sense it's a good thing to know what's
ahead of you. But after two decades I'm sure she has heard
some horror stories. And I'm sure those don't sit well with
you and result in some sleepless nights. I think that's the one
exception that I would be okay with being oblivious to the
truth.

Strong One
My grandfather was in and out of remission a few years before
he passed away. Somehow, he remained positive despite
leaving the hospital one day and answering the phone just to
hear that he had to go back again (explains the revolving

doors at hospitals). My mother must've inherited his courage as well. In her memoir, she talks about how she would draw strength from my grandfather's memory. She would also say that we gave her so much strength but, to be honest, she carried us through those many months. Some days I would forget about that putrid word cancer if it weren't for her bandana.

Dinner of Champions
From the first day she broke the news to us, my Mom always said that things would be "business as usual." That was our unofficial slogan. My mother kept a very tight circle during this time and only told close friends and family. She would only tell people if there was a reason to. Thankfully the grapevine didn't grow uncontrollably. There was no need to make a big deal out of something that people didn't need to know about. Many family members helped whenever they could, and we continued our lives of organized chaos. I clearly remember one night, in particular, when my aunt made dinner for us; it was none other than stuffed shells.

Even before this series of unfortunate coincidences, stuffed shells were far from my favorite meal. The ricotta-filled pasta went from a dinner I could muscle through to an unbearable dish. Along with the agonizing taste of the Italian cheese come the memories of my mother's diagnosis, chemotherapy, radiation, and everything in between. But there is the sweet aftertaste of the words survivor, remission, and cancer free.

-    TYLER P. BRISBOIS

· preface ·

In December 2006 I was diagnosed with Stage II invasive ductal breast cancer shortly after my forty first birthday. As you can imagine, it was a tumultuous time even as my prognosis was good. The next eight months were occupied with seventy-five appointments that included eight 'rounds' of intravenous chemotherapy, a lumpectomy and thirty-four radiation treatments in an unfamiliar world.

My husband Brian and I met in nursing school in the 1980's and have three amazing children. Travis and Tyler were in high school and Mackenzie a sixth grader at that time. Our house was bustling to say the least. Time stood still for a while, but as we adopted a "business as usual" mantra, we trudged along and learned remarkable lessons about life and family.

While I didn't know what the future would hold, I completed a master's degree in nursing during treatment and started a new position as nursing faculty two weeks after treatment ended. And while friends and family asked me to write my unique perspective of a cancer patient on paper, this was never about me, although there is catharsis in writing.

The memoir *Why I Hated Pink: Confessions of a Breast Cancer Survivor* was well received and handed off from one person and nurse to another as the need arose. I have tried to keep us all afloat through humor and perspective and by being 'real.'

I took everything I could from watching my Dad as he faced leukemia with Herculean strength and dignity and tried to live by his example. He was a man who didn't want to leave my Mom, me, my four siblings, and five grandchildren at the age of fifty-five, and always made sure we were doing okay.

I miss him terribly, even twenty-three years later, and hope with every fiber of my being that we have made him proud. He is reminisced through pictures and stories to the grandchildren and great grandchildren he never had the chance to meet.

Twelve Octobers: Reflections of a Breast Cancer Survivor is a culmination of the twelve years since diagnosis and beyond. It depicts life after treatment when the world has forgotten how tired you are, while navigating life with a heightened perspective of what is important and what is disposable; always with the looming threat of recurrence or metastases.

The stories on these pages were compiled from scraps of notes I have kept about 'survivorship,' poems and phrases that resonated with me, memories of growing up as the middle child in a lively family, introspection, and gratitude. Mostly it is about gratitude as I try, but often stumble to live my best life with the most beautiful people alongside me.

I have not included every thought or experience in this brief work; it wasn't possible. I have met astonishing people along the way who would put both me and my writing to shame. I have not forgotten the sundry kindnesses bestowed on me by family, friends, colleagues, students, and strangers.

I hope I have captured the beauty of their essence.

- MARYELLEN

SAILING

It is breast cancer

As the news collapsed her sail,

The boat shifted course

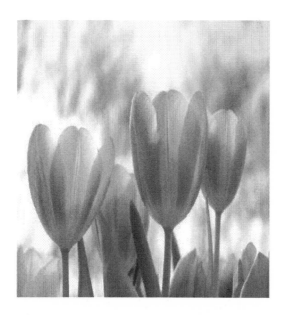

· wake ·

I remember being at our neighbor Mary's wake, kneeling next to my husband Brian at her casket. Mary had just died from an aggressive form of breast cancer after a valiant nine year 'battle.' She was dressed in light pink with a pink ribbon on her lapel. I had not officially been diagnosed with breast cancer yet, but somehow knew I had cancer growing in me that day, long before science and technology caught up with the 2.3 cm tumor (dubbed by my sister Linda as *The Fucker*) located at 1 o'clock in my left breast.

As I shifted uneasily on the kneeler, I said a prayer for Mary and her beautiful family left behind. I remember feeling strangely calm. I wondered if my own children would be as brave, valiant, and stoic as her three boys if I was the one being waked. I wondered if the community's grief would be as palpable. I also remember wondering if the line that circled outside and around the funeral parlor, into the parking lot, and down the street as far as the eye could see would be as long when I was gone.

· sand ·

I felt a thickness in my left breast by chance one morning as I lay in bed. I am not sure what prompted me to run my hand across the upper left-hand corner of my left breast, as if I knew something was there. I made an appointment with the gynecologist who soon after ordered a mammogram, ultrasound, and referral for surgical consultation.

At the appointment with the surgeon, I was told there was nothing suspicious on the recent mammogram or ultrasound, and the thickness likely due to breast density. The seasoned surgeon and new nurse practitioner (NP) were debating whether to do a fine needle aspiration (FNA) of the 'density' because I was insisting that something was wrong. While they were being 'gracious,' they asked if I wanted to have an FNA done at once to be certain. My heart was screaming "THIS ISN'T HAPPENING RIGHT NOW" (who ever would WANT a FNA?) but my head whispered, "Yes."

The decision was made. As they readied the equipment, I readied myself. The needle that pierced my skin as I looked at the stained ceiling sounded like a metal shovel striking wet beach sand. Judging by the look on the faces of the surgeon and NP, I was in trouble. I quickly got dressed, grabbed my stuff, left, and waited at home for the phone call saying I had cancer.

· intuition ·

The first inkling that something had run amok was the week of Mackenzie's (Kenzie's) First Communion four years prior. I did not feel like myself but couldn't pinpoint what was wrong. My hormones were crazy, and I was out of sorts for no reason.

The second sign my seemingly healthy body sent me was when I had time to go for a run, I didn't. It happened repeatedly. A subtle change in routine, but I cannot overestimate the importance of being in tune with ourselves and our body.

The third was the thickness in my breast. While I never made the connection at the time, these three events, coupled with the gynecologist following up on a lump for a couple of years, indicated that something was amok and later confirmed by a core biopsy and magnetic resonance imaging (MRI).

· everything changes ·

Once my suspicion was confirmed with a diagnosis
that included the size, extent, and grade of the tumor
(The *Fu**er*), lymph node involvement (none), and spread
to a different part of my body (nope); everything in my life
changed instantly, and I mean everything! Hair, food
choices, daily schedule, relationships, bra choices, energy
level, deodorant, faith, strength, outlook, skin, thought
processes, dreams and how I now looked skeptically at the
future.

Fast forward and picture yourself looking in the mirror
as a bald woman with no eyebrows who can't get out of
bed in the morning without a reveille-type call. A woman
who was forty-one years old who worked and went to
school. A wife and mother of three who had a lump in
her breast for several years. A woman who became
hyper-aware that life could change without a moment's
notice.

· news day ·

As the diagnosis and treatment plan were sorted out and marked in indelible ink on the calendar, I happened across Lauren Terrazzano, a reporter for *Newsday.* Her column, "Life, With Cancer," depicted her story with lung cancer in its terminal stage.

While her writing was sparkling, alive, and honest, she gave both hope and reality their due. I was struggling to find a positive fresh voice who wrote with humor and was close to my age. I waited for each brilliant column anxiously. I was diagnosed with breast cancer in December of 2006 and she kept me going, upright and realistic, until she passed away in May 2007 as I shifted to the radiation phase of treatment.

While her loss was a severe blow, I carried her insight and viewpoints, inspired to express myself through writing. Though I will never reach her ability to transcribe or encourage, she gave me the tremendous gift of how to live one moment at a time, and the utter catharsis of writing it all down.

· legacy ·

"If someone says your name, and it makes someone else

smile, that's a good legacy to leave."

- ROY WILLIAMS
  North Carolina Tar Heels Basketball Coach

· omnipotent ·

Even though I am mostly healthy again, I feel as if I am
racing against the clock-there is so much I want to accomplish.
I spent the first eight months of 2007 undergoing eight rounds
of chemotherapy, a sentinel node biopsy, lumpectomy, and
thirty-four radiation treatments. I thought that I knew
everything when I finished my last treatment. But I learned
that stepping back onto the tracks of life after being derailed
was difficult. Yet, every day I'm stronger and more astute than
the one before.

· brian ·

Brian and I are opposites in that I will jump in a car, hop on a plane, throw on shoes for a run, or hike in a moment's notice. Brian is a homebody who is most comfortable in the thirty-mile radius surrounding our home. He is happiest when our grown kids are all home, sitting on the front porch, playing a game of pitch with his parents around the corner, ice fishing with the guys, hunting in the fall, a poker game with his high school friends, or having a beer with his Dad (Buppa) at the sportsman's club.

Brian works as a nurse manager and is honest and kind. During the week, we dubbed him 'work Brian,' in contrast to 'weekend Brian.' 'Work' Brian is organized all day, and each evening is found ironing his clothes for the following morning, then off to bed early. 'Weekend' Brian is more laid back. On a rare occasion, weekend Brian slips into work Brian territory, and we are all grateful for it.

Brian and I find it entertaining how Travis, Tyler and Kenzie reach out to us for different things. They send Brian funny videos, gifs, or jokes. They ask me how to apply for a mortgage, write a résumé or manage a recipe. While we are opposite in our worldview, we have always been a solid team and home is a peaceful place to be.

· trav ·

As a rookie mom, Travis made life easy. He was happy, slept well, was, and remains a lover of all food. At an early age, he started talking and never stopped. We joked that he talked so much that our 'ears would bleed.' Today he is inquisitive, no nonsense and with a keen business mind.

As a child, Travis never played. He often had a toy tool belt around his waist working on building a house for his friend Emily, showing Tyler the tools on his workbench, and memorizing facts about sharks and dinosaurs with a photographic memory. He continues to build and create, works in management, and his personality remains no nonsense.

· ty ·

Tyler is the opposite of Travis, in appearance and
personality. He never slept and was my sidekick for
many years. Today he works with patients requiring
prosthetic or orthotic support. And he always keeps us
laughing.

When he was in second grade, a fire in a cold storage
building close to home killed six firefighters. Tyler rallied
the neighborhood kids and went door to door on our road,
collecting donations for the families of the lost firefighters.
His goal was that each of the six families would have a
turkey on Christmas Day. Together, they raised several
hundred dollars that was sent to the families.

· kenzie ·

Kenzie was born with a happy disposition and remains easy-going to this day. And while she is not bothered by many things, she is not a pushover. When she was three years old playing with her brothers, I heard commotion in the cellar. I found the three of them dressing her in Tyler's baseball catchers gear. She was recruited to be goalie in a pickup game of street hockey with the older neighborhood kids.

I was not very happy about this, but they begged to let her play because she was "so good." I agreed but stood watch over the game in front of the house. Kenzie had a strong performance and deflected every attempt on goal from the net. She was and remains a force.

· poetry ·

One of Kenzie's sixth grade homework assignments
was to write a poem. She decided to write about me
and asked some questions to complete the assignment.
One of the questions asked was, "What are you afraid of?"

To be honest, I was hesitant to tell her what I was afraid of:
That I'd never see her, and her brothers grow, finish high
school, attend college, get married, and raise children if
they chose to. As my only daughter, who would look after
her? Watch her babies? Just be there for her? Would I ever
see NYC, California, or Ireland? Would I grow old?

I responded that I was afraid of "heights, spiders, and
centipedes," and left the rest of it out. Only the 'heights'
part was true; the rest of the list was too long and tragic
for a middle school poem. Her poem is as follows:

~

MARYELLEN
KIND, CARING, ORGANIZED, INTELLIGENT
RELATIVE OF TRAVIS, TYLER, AND MACKENZIE
LOVER OF HER KIDS, RUNNING, AND THE BEACH
WHO FEELS HAPPY, HEALTHY, AND STRONG
WHO NEEDS FAMILY, FRIENDS, AND CARE
WHO FEARS HEIGHTS, SPIDERS, AND CENTIPEDES
WHO GIVES SUPPORT, LOVE, AND FRIENDSHIP
WHO WOULD LIKE TO SEE NYC, CALIFORNIA,
AND IRELAND
RESIDENT OF MASSACHUSETTS
BRISBOIS
~

-   MACKENZIE D. BRISBOIS

· speed demon ·

While in the throes of chemotherapy, spring had
unceremoniously arrived. I decided to walk to my in-law's
house around the corner. I needed a warm jacket, but the air
was refreshing. It had been a long winter and I felt as though
someone had put my chemo-headed brain topped with a wig
(dubbed 'the raccoon') on someone else's weary body. I
realized there was a gaping abyss between survival and
livelihood. But this day was a good one as I made my way
along.

As I rounded a bend in the road, I heard a car with a loud
muffler in the distance. We were traveling in the same
direction, but clearly at different speeds. I turned in time to
realize the elderly driver hadn't seen me and I had to jump
into the woods to get out of her way. She was so close to me
that the car hit my hand as she sped past. I gained my
composure, straightened out the raccoon, stepped into the
road and continued to my destination.

Minutes later, she turned the car around and gave me hell for
throwing something at her car, muttering something about
"kids these days." As I described how she almost hit me with
her car, she told me to "pay more attention."

At that time, I was on high alert to every little nuance in my
body, overprotective of myself. I never thought an elderly
woman speeding along a country road might have been the
death of me.

· haircuts and gum ·

After I lost my hair, two weeks after the first chemotherapy
infusion, I continued to shampoo my bald head every day.
I even caught myself absentmindedly tucking the 'hair'
behind my right ear out of habit. It always made me smile,
as old ways are hard to break. Thankfully, I lost my hair
but not my sense of humor.

As you can imagine, the first hair cut after chemotherapy
ends is a glorious occasion. It seemed like a major turning
point and another thing in life that I had never given a
second thought. I was astonished that it hurt my head to
have a vigorous shampoo and cut. It was as if each strand
of new hair was attached by a pin to my head. The
anticipated bliss of this event was overshadowed by
the nerve endings in my scalp screaming in unison.

I didn't have the heart to say anything to my new hair
stylist because it was a celebration, damn it! I remained
hesitant to let my hair grow past the length it was before
Brian buzzed it off one Sunday morning. But I must admit
that it still hasn't made it past my shoulders as the years
march on.

I was also looking forward to chewing cinnamon gum
post chemotherapy. I had sores in my mouth from
treatment and missed chewing my favorite flavored gum.
However, more than a decade later, cinnamon flavored
gum still burns my tongue, and spearmint gum doesn't
quite take its place.

· quitters ·

I knew I was considered back to 'normal' when two things happened: The housecleaning that my husband and three children had been doing weekly for eight months suddenly came to a screeching halt the precise moment I finished radiation therapy.

The second, but equally blatant, sign was when Travis voiced that he liked me better when I had chemotherapy because I was a "lot more mellow then." Travis could be relieved because it didn't mean I was the same person after treatment than I was before. A well needed break from the fact that I ran a tight ship was well noted that day! I think we would all be happy with the change.

· living well ·

"The secret to living well and longer is: eat half,

walk double, laugh triple, and love without measure."

- TIBETAN PROVERB

· leo ·

My godfather, Uncle Leo, used to play 'catch' with us whenever we visited my grandmother. We would bring our baseball gloves with us for this reason. He wore white shoes and had a DA (duck's ass) haircut from the 1950's; both of which continue to this day. He and my godmother, Auntie Carolyn, were always kind to me, especially at birthdays, and when I had my tonsils removed as a child.

When I was five years old, Uncle Leo mentioned I would be a good nurse. From that moment on, I decided I would pursue the profession of nursing. I have never looked back and truly believe it is the best profession. Shortly after I completed my PhD, I saw them both at a family funeral and recalled our conversation regarding nursing to him. He didn't remember saying that to me. It's funny to think that one comment formulated many of the choices I made to pursue a career in nursing. I am grateful for that.

· four things ·

For as long as I can remember, I have wanted to accomplish four things: run a marathon, learn to swim, play the piano, and write a book. I am not sure if I will ever run a marathon, but in running two half-marathons, I count them as a full marathon, and *triple dog dare you* to challenge that one.

I did legitimately learn to swim in my late thirties with my sister Erin when training for a triathlon. Every time I struggled into a one-piece navy-blue Speedo, and slid into the chilly water, I immediately had a flashback to the only other swimming lesson I had.

· swimming and other lessons ·

As a wary fifth grader, I boarded a yellow school bus with my class bound for the Girl's Club across town. When we disembarked the bus, I slowly walked toward the building, permission slip tight in hand. We were led down a long corridor with pale green walls to the locker room.

The lifeguard on duty handed us each a bathing suit she pulled from a trough of bleach-like solution with silver tongs. Wrestling the wet bathing suit on in front of classmates, trying to keep myself covered, was impossible.

We left the locker room in tandem, smelling like bleach, to the pool area. Some of us swam laps and the rest of us were in line to jump off the diving board. The board looked to be about four miles above the water; we were expected to jump in! I arrived at the top of the ladder and wobbled to the board's edge, panicked, crawled back to the ladder, and climbed past each girl waiting her turn to jump.

As I was going through treatment, these memories flooded my brain. But this time, I was determined to *jump*, leaving my ten-year-old self behind on the diving board.

· piano lessons ·

I have long desired to learn how to play the piano.
I played the violin in grammar school and in a city-wide
orchestra through the eighth grade. I received a keyboard
from my sister Erin, that quietly sits untouched in the attic.
I can only hope I am more successful with this goal than
jumping off diving boards.

· writing a book ·

I have always loved to write, but quite frankly, never imagined any book I might write would be about an experience with breast cancer. But *Why I Hated Pink* was kicked around in my brain before I penned it, and *Twelve Octobers* is no different. Sometimes our ambitions, though seemingly unattainable, are realized differently than anticipated in the form of something far greater than imagined.

· on writing ·

"I write. The longer I live, the more convinced I've become that I cultivate my truest self in this one way."

- TOM CHIARELLA
  Permission to publish the quote has been requested

· eileen ·

As *Why I Hated Pink* became available, I received many messages of support. One of my favorites was from a middle and high school classmate of my brother who wrote that she read the entire book standing at her kitchen sink. Since then, we correspond daily, sending messages and memes back and forth. Although she lives across the country, we are quite determined and equipped to solve the problems of the world.

· down the hatch ·

One memory of my father remains after being diagnosed at the age of fifty with Stage IV leukemia. Soon after, he started chemotherapy by mouth with hope of remission.

The first day of this regime, he described standing in front of the kitchen sink in a suit and tie and filling a tall glass with water. It took three valiant attempts to place the pills in his mouth and rinse them down. He then left for work. The following morning, it took two tries. On the third day he was good to go.

He was hesitant to tell his co-workers and supervisor about the cancer. He pulled the charade off for many months, until missing work due to low white blood cell counts. Even then, he only told a select few.

· tamoxifen ·

Phase four of treatment for me consisted of five years of
Tamoxifen by mouth. Tamoxifen is used to treat hormone-
receptor positive, early, locally advanced, and metastatic
breast cancer. I was prescribed Tamoxifen instead of
aromatase inhibitors (AIs) because I was still getting my
period, although less frequently.

I can't say that taking my first dose of Tamoxifen was
anything like my father taking a mouthful of pills at the sink.
But I started the first of 1,825 doses on August sixth, the
thirteenth anniversary of my dad's passing.

I still cannot differentiate what effects I had from
chemotherapy, radiation and/or Tamoxifen. I *do* know that
my brain and vision were *partly cloudy*, monstrous *charlie
horses* kept me awake at night, I gained weight, and had
"ketchup legs."

Ketchup legs were coined by my nursing school buddies
(NSBs) Cathy, Monique (Moke) and Francie to describe the
feeling that the blood flow in one's legs is as thick as ketchup.
This 'condition' is most common after a long day of work at
the hospital or, in this case, while on Tamoxifen.

· bonus prize ·

As the five-year mark since diagnosis passed unceremoniously, and I received a clean bill of health, I stopped taking Tamoxifen per protocol. Some effects I experienced waxed and waned, making it difficult to discern their cause.

Five months later, after meeting with the oncologist, a published research study recommended a second five-year course of Tamoxifen could reduce the chance of recurrence in pre-menopausal women. In post-menopausal women, AIs were the drug of choice for the extended timeframe.

Still premenopausal, I received a new prescription for Tamoxifen. I didn't pick it up at the pharmacy for a week or two or three, because I had been feeling more like my 'old' self and enjoyed being reunited with her. I finally started on February 6th, my mother's birthday, and six months from the day I completed the first round.

I was ten or so doses into the new prescription when it felt as if all two hundred and six bones in my body were exploding. I didn't recall this happening the first time (I don't think I would have forgotten *that*). I called the oncologist for some advice. She recommended that I change the time of the dose to bedtime. I hung up the phone, shaking my head, thinking that the sensation of my bones exploding at night wouldn't be much better, but I did follow her advice. After a few nights of fireworks, it all settled down. The second phase of Tamoxifen breezed by and I finished on my mother's seventy-eighth birthday with little fanfare and all bones intact.

· nana ·

I was blessed with two amazing grandmothers, and one great- grandmother. They were 'old' school in the sense that they never wore pants or drove a car. But they were ahead of themselves in that they set the bar high for their future generations and loved us unconditionally.

My paternal grandmother, Nana (Margaret), was a spitfire who worked in the school department in a big city. She could type faster than anyone I ever knew and would be horrified by my two-finger typing style and pirate-like swearing. She was also a whiz at shorthand, which I never quite grasped, but was amazed by. We spent countless hours with her and my grandfather until he passed. My memories are immeasurable; I most recall her pride in her grandchildren. It still resonates in me.

Nana also wore a *hot pink* feather hat shaped like an upside-down bird nest. When it was raining, she covered it with a clear rain hat tied under her chin. I can still picture Nana (singing off key) and the seven of us (five of whom were fidgeting) filling a pew each Sunday in church, with the Finnegan family bounding in late to fill the pew in front of us.

While in nursing school, my NSBs and I were crossing from the dorm to the hospital when Nana drove by us in the passenger seat of a car. My roommate Cathy yelled, "Look at that lady's HAT!" I quietly replied that she was my grandmother. At first, they didn't believe me, but she was later dubbed *Grandma Hat* after I convinced them I was telling the truth.

From my grandfather Jack, I inherited the habit of writing words, phrases, poems, and ideas on scraps of paper like the ones I found lying on his desk and end tables. It was like an unplanned scavenger hunt for me to uncover. This is just how I organize my ideas, even though it may look like chaos from the outside. He also survived a plane crash, but thankfully that isn't a genetic predisposition.

· grammie ·

My maternal grandmother and grandfather lived an hour
away. We saw them less often than my Dad's parents.
Grammie (Sophie) always waited on the front porch for us to
arrive. We were a lively bunch of five kids hopping out of an
overcrowded station wagon. And since I had perpetual
motion sickness, she always asked if I had been sick, as if my
green pallor didn't give it away. She called each of her twenty-
nine grandchildren *Cookie*, but somehow made us feel like we
were the only *Cookie* in the universe.

One Easter Sunday after dinner was devoured by my cousins,
aunts, and uncles, I decided to help with the dishes and was
standing in front of her white porcelain sink. I was welcomed
into the throng of women, even though I was just a young
teenager; my grandmother clearly in charge. She looked at me
and said, "Cookie, grab a towel and dry some dishes and
remember: don't ever take any wooden nickels."

I can still picture my grandfather Stephen sitting at the head of
the kitchen table with a hot pot of tea in front of him each time
we visited. The first thing I do when my feet hit the ground,
after making the bed, is put tea on to start the day. He also
published a book titled *Western Massachusetts History* in 1970.
Each of us are truly pieces of those who came before us,
woven together.

· grandma ·

My maternal great grandmother (Mary) was born in 1883 and emigrated to the United States (U.S.) at the turn of the twentieth century. She was strong and beautiful and stood barely five feet tall.

She and my great grandfather (Louis) lived well into their nineties and were married over seventy years. They welcomed each of us with open arms but I'm quite sure Grandma couldn't tell her great grandchildren apart. She would ask, "Who is your mother?"and we'd laugh and tell her who we belonged to.

I started to think a lot about the impact my grandparents and great grandparents had on me. Their traditions, love of family, strength and wisdom are sewn to my heart. I have dreamed about growing old, although I can't imagine it happening. If I *do* grow old, I aspire to be like Kate Blackwell, matriarch in Sidney Sheldon's *Master of the Game.*

If I become a grandmother along the way, I'd like to be called *Mia.* Some of my favorite people call me Mia. In German, it means 'we are we' or 'we are who we are;' in Italian, it simply means 'mine.'

· women ·

"Women hold up half the sky."

- MAO ZEDONG
  Now in the public domain

· #$@&%! sweater ·

Before every Christmas holiday, my two older siblings
(Karen and Joe) and I would rummage through the house
to see what gifts our parents had tucked away for us.
We were so intent in knowing what we were getting ahead
of time that we went to great lengths to find out. Most years,
we left no stone unturned in the search. Some years, we
would unwrap, then rewrap each gift, so we would not be
caught.

During one December escapade, my sister and I found a
beautiful sweater that we each claimed as our own but
had to wait it out. When Christmas morning *finally* arrived,
the sweater (meticulously rewrapped by yours truly) had
Karen's name scrolled on the package. I was *devastated*. I
learned that things weren't always as they seemed, and
while waiting is difficult, good things come to those who are
patient…or so I'm told.

· virtue ·

Patience is a virtue that dates to the fifth century, but it is not one that I possess. Everyone who knows me, is fully aware of this tragic flaw. But I disagree.

I *am* patient in waiting for a project or relationship to unfold in its own time.

I *am* patient when I could be angry but try to move on instead.

I *am* patient when someone is trying to understand something that doesn't come easily to them.

I *am trying to be more patient* as I age, because wisdom and patience complement one another, and I am wanting to be both.

Photo Credit: graceandgrind.wordpress.com

I am *not* patient with myself.

I am *not* patient with drama, untruthfulness, or laziness.

I am *not* patient when being taken advantage of.

· jewelry box ·

The following year after the sweater debacle and Thanksgiving holiday, my father began making a wooden jewelry box for *someone* in the cellar under the cloak of darkness. Those were the glory days when hot pink was my favorite color. I had known he was working on *something* at his work bench and even snuck a peek at the unfinished gift (old habits die hard). Only *this* time, I thought it was for my younger sister Linda.

On Christmas morning, the beautiful and perfect wooden jewelry box lined with pink velvet was *mine*. Mine! It even had a tiny lock and key designed to keep my prying siblings out. The sight of that chest, and the smell of sawdust instantly bring me back to my childhood, even today.

· renew ·

A former colleague and friend Barbara reached out to me
when she was diagnosed with breast cancer. We spoke
back and forth, and I'd send a card of support along the way.

When I was going through chemotherapy, she sent me a
handmade prayer shawl for comfort. When she was at the
end of her chemo, I sent a card with this message: Barbara,
so happy to hear you are finished with this part of your
journey! Now it's time to:

Reawaken	Revitalize
Rejoice	Restock
Revive	Resume
Rejuvenate	Regain
Regroup	Replenish
Replenish	Recreate
Renew	Revel
Reaffirm	Regenerate

It was a message for Barbara, but really for all of us, to take
time to heal and process what transpired. It felt like crawling
out of a dark cave into bright sunlight without knowing if
you would have to climb back into the darkness for another
go around.

· environment ·

While preparing dinner one night, the local news on television caught my attention. The newscaster was covering a story about a chemical plant that dumped toxic dyes into the local river for almost one hundred years. The Environmental Protection Agency (EPA) made a link between the dye in the river to cases of sarcoma in young men who lived and attended school near the plant.

My father had worked a quarter of a mile from the chemical plant for twenty-nine years. When Dad was diagnosed with leukemia, his oncologist was certain he had been exposed to something in the environment that caused a gene-environment reaction. I can assure you that my father never missed a day of work until he was hospitalized from complications of leukemia treatment that necessitated an early retirement. At best count, he spent over 7,500 days at that workplace.

In my master's program, I completed a project on the history of the chemical company and the negative effect it had on the local community. One young man who developed sarcoma brought the story into the forefront, prompting the EPA investigation. I never met Kevin Kane as he passed away in 1998, but I met his mother when I was invited to 'kick off' an *American Cancer Society Relay for Life* event in the town where Kevin grew up, and Dad worked to support his family.

I later had an opportunity to teach an environmental health course to registered nurses. Life is full of serendipitous moments if you keep an eye out for them.

· teaching the teacher ·

After completing a master's degree, I began teaching nursing full-time at a local university. I had a two-week reprieve between the end of treatment and the start of the fall semester. I was just out of the bald stage after giving up my wig (the raccoon) in late July, had no eyebrows or eyelashes yet, but was in full swing the minute I unlocked my office door, still unsure if this was one of my best ideas.

I apparently had something to prove, was in desperate need of some normalcy, and somehow, after all these years, still wanting to make my father proud. My determination was boundless; my energy level not so much. I taught Chronic Illness, Community Health and Leadership in Nursing courses over my six years there. I had two brilliant mentors who taught me by example and challenged me; as did hundreds of students who continue to impart their wisdom via social media or over a cup of joe.

I also enrolled in a PhD in nursing program after the first year of teaching. I had become preoccupied with health disparities that existed in treatment outcomes and life expectancy between a white woman with breast cancer and a Latina woman. I have always been a champion of the underdog since grammar school recess, and this seemed like interesting and meaningful research for my dissertation. It was during this semester in the PhD program that I wrote *Why I Hated Pink: Confessions of a Breast Cancer Survivor*. It had been kicking around my brain and I desperately needed to put it on paper to move on and learn everything I could about health disparities and research.

· doctor nurse ·

The young Latina women whom I interviewed for my dissertation were courageous, lively, and honest in answering the personal questions I asked them about the impact of breast cancer on them, especially with their experience of chemotherapy-induced premature menopause. I was awarded a doctoral degree scholarship from the *American Cancer Society* for my work, no doubt one of my proudest achievements.

I spoke to women from across the country who shared a common vision of being well enough to work and care for their families and themselves despite the barriers they faced. I never met any of these women (like the 'pinkies') but their voices became part of my soul and I carry them with me in a spirit of camaraderie and deep respect. Again, the nursing professors and mentors were brilliant and taught me many skills, but from the study participants stories and grit, I learned the most.

I graduated with my PhD on National Cancer Survivor Day; much like my master's degree graduation being on Mother's Day. With the stars somehow aligned, I accepted a new teaching position at a university, some sixty miles from home.

· college bound ·

While enrolled in school, Travis went off to college, completing both a baccalaureate and master's degree. Soon after, Tyler followed, accomplishing the same. Kenzie finished her undergraduate degree in Economics and enrolled in a nursing program. As Brian and I are both nurses, we are thrilled with her decision. She played college softball for a season and my days back on the road resumed. Brian also completed his master's degree with little fanfare. We spent more money on printer ink and paper than groceries some weeks, but everyone was working hard creating their own path.

When first diagnosed with breast cancer, I had made the grandiose announcement to Brian and the kids that our household would run in a 'business as usual' fashion. This blip in time would *never* be an excuse for slipping grades or poor behavior. I never imagined how seriously they would take this message to heart that was mostly intended to save me from my rapidly crumbling self.

The years of high school athletics, proms, drivers' licenses, first loves, homework, and worrying about each of them passed quickly. And the college years sped doubly fast with packing them up to live in the dorms, keeping tired cars up and running, leasing apartments, the telling of stories I never wanted to hear, and shaping their futures.

· uncertainty ·

Damocles Syndrome is the name sometimes given to the
fear that cancer will return. The name comes from the
idea that fear of recurrence can feel as if the sword of
Damocles hangs over one's head, suspended by a thin
thread. According to the story, Damocles was playing up
to the king to switch places with him, as he (Damocles) felt
worthier of the crown than the unhappy king. When the
king agreed, Damocles sat in the king's throne, only to
realize that King Dionysius II had placed a sword above
the throne held up by a single thread of a horse's tail.
Damocles begged the king to leave the throne as he
didn't want the danger associated with the position as he
now feared for his life (dictionary.com; The History Channel,
2016).

If someone is said to have the Sword of Damocles
hanging over their head, it means they are in a situation
in which something very bad could happen to them at
any time (Collins English Dictionary). To me, the
'syndrome' is synonymous with the nursing concept of
uncertainty, or a situation in which something is not
known, or certain. Uncertainty is likely to occur in a
person who is diagnosed with cancer (or other
life-threatening illness) on some level for the duration
of their life.

For me, uncertainty lifts its ugly 'sword' every six months
with follow up appointments, or when I have an ache or
pain that doesn't go away. There is no expiration date with
fear of recurrence.

· my friend ·

"Oh, my friend, it's not what they take away from you

that counts - it's what you do with what you have left."

- HUBERT HUMPHREY
  38th Vice-President of the United States
  Stated following cancer surgery in 1976

· garden ·

A few summers after treatment, I decided that I would
love to have a vegetable garden. We had a garden for
many years. What no one knew was that I enthusiastically
cherished everything living, and a garden was no exception.

Brian found a spot in the backyard and bought some loam.
Tyler planted tomatoes, cucumbers, peppers, chives, and
summer squash. The garden thrived despite my lack of a
green thumb, and I enjoyed the vegetables. Tyler became
adept at making fresh salsa by the gallon. And while he
didn't know the joy I felt watching the garden (but not
the weeds) grow, it made that summer much brighter.

We continued to have a garden each year until last
summer, because I was traveling to Barcelona for work,
caring for my beloved aunt, and Travis and Ashley's
wedding was approaching in July. Tyler, however,
did plant a splendid garden at the home he now shares
with Emily, his future bride.

· dreamer ·

"I've got dreams in hidden places and extra smiles

for when I'm blue."

-    AUTHOR UNKNOWN
     And Greatly Appreciated

· jane ·

As the word of *Why I Hated Pink* spread, I took part in several book signings. I loved making new friends and seeing old ones. I was always surprised by who stopped by to offer support or share a kind word. Dad's cousin, Franny, and her daughter, Colleen were two of the first in line. I hadn't seen either of them for many years, except through Facebook. My colleague Jerry from the university swung by, followed by Katie and a steady stream of people I didn't know.

One person I didn't recognize stopped to say hello. She introduced herself as Jane. It took me a minute to realize that right before my eyes stood JANE! We hugged, and I became overwhelmed with joy and a thousand other emotions.

Jane was a co-worker of Brian's when I was first diagnosed. A breast cancer survivor herself, she would send along 'tips' of what to expect and how to deal with what was coming next in the most positive way. These tips were relayed to me through Brian, and *every single day* for over a year, the first thing I asked Brian when he arrived home from work was, "Did you happen to see Jane today? If so, does she have any new messages for me?"

There are no words to explain the gratitude I had and continue to have for Jane. She literally saved me. Tears are welling in my eyes as I type with two fingers.

· collateral damage ·

During a very vital work meeting, dressed in a favorite dress, I happened to look down only to realize my breasts were completely different sizes. It's not so much that they were not symmetrical, but more so that I never noticed it before.

While trying to pay close attention to the meeting proceedings I tried to contain my laughter. I bit my lip and covered my mouth with my hand but couldn't contain the smirk plastered on my face. I'm not sure if it was the dress I had on that emphasized the difference or not.

I play a mind game with myself to put my life in perspective and repeatedly, it works. This is how it goes: Say I'm in a car accident and my car is totaled. I think, *Well, at least I'm okay and no one got hurt.* Or I have a stressful day at work and think, *Well, at least I'm lucky to have a job.* After the meeting adjourned, I thought to myself, *Well, at least I have my breasts and a warped sense of humor.* A few days later, my 'favorite' dress was quietly dropped off at a local thrift shop.

· pretending ·

Sometimes I think if things or events don't directly

affect us, it is easier to pretend they don't exist

anywhere in the world.

· personal care products ·

Brian's colleague Jane informed Brian that putting aloe gel on the radiated area immediately after treatment would improve the condition of my skin. I also learned to use deodorant 'crystals' instead of regular deodorant and to use soap and lotions with no fragrance in them.

When I gave up on reading the literature regarding the side effects of each medication and chemo-therapeutic agent I was given along the way, I was drawn to environmental risk factors associated with cancer. This was of interest to me as my father's leukemia was related to his workplace and I had no genetic predisposition to the disease.

I read extensively and discovered there might be a link between the personal care products and cleaning products used in our households and cancer. An endocrine disruption seems to be where things go astray.

"The average U.S. woman uses 12 personal care products and/or cosmetics a day, containing 168 different chemicals" (Environmental Working Group). Men use fewer chemicals, but still place 85 chemicals directly on their bodies every day. Many chemicals are unregulated because of 'trade secrets' and lack of oversight, with little understanding of how the numerous chemicals in each product interact with each other and impact our health. However, there is now a wealth of information regarding what chemicals to avoid, and a plethora of products on the market that have fewer chemicals than the major brands used for years.

· fenway ·

We moved into a new home across town two years before
my diagnosis. It was a good move, but we were leaving the
best neighbors and wonderful place for the kids to grow.
Our dog Shadow didn't make the move with us, because she
was advanced in age and very ill.

The kids really wanted a new puppy after we settled in.
One day, much to Brian's dismay, we brought home a
Labradoodle and named him Fenway. While my intent
was for the kids to have a companion in our new home,
I never anticipated that Fenway would be a huge support
to me when I was going through treatment. He would keep
me company and was always a willing partner if I needed a
nap. He was nonjudgmental if that nap lasted a considerable
amount of time while the kids were in school.

We lost Fenway in March after 13 ½ years of magnificence.
The kids all swung over to pay their due to a dog who was
more like a friend, with a heart as big as his head.

· first lady ·

"You gain strength, courage and confidence by every

experience in which you really stop to look fear in the face."

- ELEANOR ROOSEVELT
  First Lady of the United States
  Now in the public domain

· eulogies ·

My paternal grandmother *(Grandma Hat)* passed away
the spring before Brian and I were married. I found a poem
I thought fitting and asked if I could read it at her funeral.
I have always had a sense that memories of places and
people must be immortalized, whether through photos,
bringing up memories in conversations with loved ones,
or on paper.

I was mostly a quiet kid, except for the million questions
I asked my parents every day, and when I was with my
brother and sisters. I swear my mother sent me to
kindergarten at four years of age because I asked her so
many questions; she has never denied this. I wanted to
know how things *worked* and loved to 'work' alongside
my father in his workshop in the cellar or listen to
conversations he had with grown-ups.

When he became very ill with months to live, I started to
jot down things that reminded me of him. I never wanted
him (especially him!) to be forgotten and felt inclined to
write a 'tribute' of sorts to him that ended up being the
eulogy at his funeral. It started out like this, "My father
hated eulogies, but being his middle child, I somehow
feel entitled..."

His eulogy was well received and since then, I have
written and given several eulogies for loved ones at
funeral masses. Our beloved Fenway was also eulogized
recently, but on Facebook.

· shy me ·

I outgrew my shyness in high school and haven't stopped talking since (sorry Travis)! And though I was shy, I have never minded formally speaking in front of a crowd, if I'm prepared, and I can wing an impromptu discussion if necessary. I believe that I am an introverted extrovert as I need time to think and refuel, but a nap or a run usually do the trick.

· don't you forget about me ·

I also have an overwhelming desire or desperate need to leave a legacy. I struggle with finding my 'calling' beyond nursing, teaching, and breast cancer. I don't know where my life is going; this is mostly thrilling, but somewhat daunting.

I don't want to be forgotten which sounds immensely selfish. But whatever happens down the road, please keep me where the light is and in your heart.

· wisdom ·

"Love is something that you can leave behind when you die.

It's that powerful."

\- JOHN (FIRE) LAME DEER

· advocacy ·

There is an unwritten culture among cancer patients in
that they have an affinity to give back to society or to those
patients diagnosed after them. Although this sense of
advocacy is strong, it is often difficult to find one's place
in a bottomless sea of mammoth agencies and foundations.
While I never was inspired to join a support group during
treatment, I did attend one at a local YWCA during the
dissertation stage of my PhD to be sure I had data
regarding chemotherapy-induced premature menopause
from every angle possible.

I felt more comfortable offering my limited time and energy
to local groups vested in supporting women and men
through advocacy, education, and closing the gaps
(assistance with meals, bills, transportation) that many
cancer patients face. Being an advocate for the
environment, I realized that the pink ribbon was placed
on many items, with the promise of proceeds going to
breast cancer research. While this can be an admirable
charge, corporations use their notoriety to *pinkwash*' or
support breast cancer causes to promote themselves or
their services. There is a sense among many breast cancer
patients that we are being used to support corporate
greed.

This ongoing and widespread practice was and is difficult
for me to wrap my brain around, but instead of supporting
their questionable motives, I became interested in
The Gloria Gemma Foundation, *Dresses that Cure*, The *15-40
Connection* and *Pink Revolution* in my 'backyard.' Their work
is extraordinary and far reaching.

On a small scale, I have had the privilege of speaking to
different community groups (schools, workplaces, breast

cancer organizations, etc.) about my experience, the need for prevention and reducing cancer risk, the impact of environment, and writing workshops. On a grander scale, I have had the opportunity to speak to larger crowds to kick off events for the American Cancer Society and discuss my dissertation research at national nursing conferences. It has been an exhilarating whirlwind, but one that can be emotional and sap my energy.

To lighten it up, I typically open with a disclaimer saying something like, "I can get choked up telling my story. There are two problems with this. The first is that I never know when it will happen. The second is that it ruins my badass image." Surprisingly enough, I often get a laugh at that moment. When I *do* get choked up, it helps us all get through.

I would never have made it through cancer treatment without scores of people who came to my aid, led the way out of the darkness and brought me back from the brink. I hope my voice has helped others along the way.

· october ·

Oh October!

Once the start of the most splendid season of vibrant

colors; nowadays a canvas of pink.

We look to it as a time to mend something broken,

throwing money and hope into air as if it will vanish.

When it never had to appear and perpetuate.

· waning strength ·

There are many 'things' a cancer patient loses. To me, physical strength and energy were the hardest to see evaporate before my eyes. Truth be told, I am grateful that regardless of these losses, I was spared from having extensive surgery or debilitating effects of treatment.

I went from training for and running half marathons and completing a triathlon, to being unable to run a mile without stopping thirty-four times. Before cancer, I would run barefoot on a treadmill on the steepest incline for six, seven, or eight miles at a time without a second thought.

I so missed the ruthless second wind that got me through a lot of things in my overbooked pre-cancer life. I miss the second wind less than strength because it has made me stop for the day at a more reasonable hour and improved my quality of life. The good things that endured were determination and resilience which helped cut the losses. And still, I run.

· twice a year ·

Since crossing the treatment finish line, I have continued
to have follow up appointments every six months, and
now yearly. While there is trepidation as each appointment
nears, I am further away from December 22nd in 2006 when
I heard the words, *"You have cancer."*

There have been many threats of recurrence dodged along
the way, including suspicious cysts (in both breasts) that
warranted an ultrasound and/or biopsy, endometrial
thickening (also biopsied), ovarian cysts, a numb left
shoulder (from sentinel node biopsy) that necessitated
x-rays and a CT scan to rule out metastases, and physical
therapy to manage. When I asked how long the numbness
in my shoulder might last, the oncologist stated she wasn't
sure, but eventually "patients stop complaining about it."
And on that day, I stopped complaining about it too.

The veins in my right arm are sclerosed and thin like
spaghetti but strong as steel from chemotherapy;
challenging for phlebotomists during blood draws.
Chronic neuropathy and plantar fasciitis round out the
package deal, but again, things could be worse, and I
choose to ignore them.

· mri ·

Every six months, I have either a mammogram or MRI to screen for recurrence or metastasis. In addition to Brian knowing, I often tell only one or two friends about upcoming testing. To me, it seems unfair to get everyone hyped up for no reason.

As I did with screening appointments during the diagnosis phase, I often go by myself to make the awkward climb onto the MRI machine in a backward hospital gown, with breasts exposed. This makes even the strongest person diminish to a weakling the instant the strings of the unbending gown are tied.

Six months later, it's mammogram time. And while a mammogram is never a comfortable procedure, it is doubly sore when an astute technician manages to squish every bit of flesh from clavicle to bottom of rib cage into the machine and reduce it to the size of a pancake. Then, repeat MRI six months later.

· stuck ·

Because I have received good news post mammogram and MRI screenings, it is always easier to let one or two 'knowing friends' that my results are negative. And while it isn't about me, but instead of the impact of recurrence and the stopping of life on a dime, I always send good news regarding results with an addendum that they're *stuck with me,* at least for a while.

If I do get the news of recurrence or metastasis one day, the message will begin with 'Hello darkness, my old friend.' Then you will know.

· bloom ·

'Bloom where you are planted' the old saying goes,

But if you find yourself wilting in time or space,

Fear not and pollinate,

As would the bewitching rose.

· new office ·

The new teaching position I accepted at the university would allow me the opportunity to learn and expand my novice research and scientific writing skills. Because it was also a state university, I was able to transfer hundreds of sick hours I had accrued, in case I needed them.

As an assistant professor on a dreaded tenure track, the next five years of my life were outlined in intricate detail regarding scholarship (research) and professional activities, teaching, advising and service requirements. I was ready for the challenge, even without a second wind. My sister-in-law, Corinne, gave me a print for my old office that I hung in my new office. It had brought me good luck before, and I hoped for more of the same.

The commute is long and sometimes tedious, but I make playlists of favorite songs, to not be distracted by radio commercials and dials along the way. Kenzie was living away at college, so I didn't feel I would be missing her activities as in high school, but I sure did miss her. I would play *Ain't No Sunshine* by Bill Withers on repeat. I began to enjoy the down time in the car back and forth to campus, always with songs blaring and me singing along at the top of my lungs and a little off key, like Grandma Hat.

· travel ·

Six weeks into the new position and the fall semester, the department chair called a meeting. At first, I thought something was wrong, but since she was incredible at providing support and answering my million questions, I calmed down.

She asked me if I was interested in bringing a group of students to Haiti the following spring; a tradition since the 2010 earthquake struck. The former professor had retired, and the opportunity was mine for the taking. Of course, I said "yes" without hesitation.

A couple of weeks later, the Chair called another meeting asking if I was interested in traveling to the Azores, Portugal with a delegation of senators, congressional representatives, and university officials. My role was to explore the possibility of starting a nursing student exchange with the university there; something that had been in discussion for twenty-seven years. I jumped at the opportunity. These two improbable opportunities facilitated the capacity for me to work with underserved and vulnerable people a hundred-fold.

· new normal ·

There is a notion floating out there that cancer patients adjust to a *new normal* post treatment that is exemplified by a life full of unicorns, endless sunny days, rainbows, parades, and champagne fountains bubbling over from our bathtubs.

For me, it was instead a time of relief, loneliness, and profound introspection. The shift to normal (whatever that is) was not as straightforward as the clear delineation of life before cancer (BC) and after cancer (AC) that can be narrowed down to a precise moment in time. *Nothing* is normal AC. Nothing.

But there is a robust desire from inside to move on, resume prior activities and schedules, and toss away anything that resembles drama or bullshit. A person living BC to AC has time on their hands to put things in perspective and do everything but take the act of living for granted. And if you find us on the outside looking in pensively, please be patient. We carry the heavy and unspoken burden about when our gig on earth will be up and if we are doing enough to make up for when the inevitable happens.

· flair ·

"I would have liked to have gone out with a bit more flair,

but I feel I can die with dignity.

I don't think it matters how long you live, so long as you

can say: I've got everything out of life."

- MARGARET MOTH
  Acclaimed photojournalist CNN documentary 2010

· twelve octobers ·

Once I realized the 2.3 cm lump in my left breast was trying to kick my ass, and subsequent treatment did indeed kick it, I needed to put the whole thing in some perspective.

Calculator in hand, I realized that this October, twelve years will have passed since I first palpated thickness in my breast. Twelve wild, crazy Octobers with more highs than lows, laughter than tears and with a zest for life that exhausts most people.

So here goes: 53 birthdays x 12 months/8 months of treatment = 636 months/8 months = 0.01257862 *or* 1.25% of my life was spent in treatment mode.

A mere 1.25%. In full realization that time is the ultimate currency, I am a *very* wealthy woman.

· pieces of the puzzle ·

At birth, each of us hold a piece of the universe's puzzle in our heart, mind, and tiny fist. Each path is pre-destined but shaped through thought, intent, and action. I can assure you with certainty that no one in the delivery room (or waiting outside for the news) can anticipate which puzzle piece is in the newborn's hand, or where it will fit. Being open to possibility and potential in life is paramount.

By most accounts, my 'forties' were amazing, except for that short blip in time. I had many opportunities, met new people, changed the course of my career, and traveled. I also learned to say 'no' to things not meant for me and embrace what was. And my fifties are even more validating. I'm happy being me.

· no regrets ·

"Live with intention. Walk to the edge. Listen hard.

Practice wellness. Play with abandon. Laugh. Choose

with no regret. Appreciate your friends. Continue to learn.

Do what you love. Live as if this is all there is."

- MARY ANNE RADMACHER
  Permission to publish the poem has been requested

· summit plummet ·

The entire Brisbois clan (15 strong) was vacationing at Walt
Disney World many years ago. Brian, sister in law Corinne,
and I decided to ride the Summit Plummet high speed
waterslide that boasts a 12-story drop in a 360-foot-long run.

There was more than one bad decision that occurred. The
first being I am terrified of heights. We climbed up countless
stairs to reach the 'summit.' Brian went first, and I was next
(must have drawn the short straw). I sat at the top of the slide,
grabbed the bar, looked down and FROZE. Corinne was right
behind me waiting her turn, encouraging me to GO without
looking down. I could hear her but was immobile.

After I started breathing again, it became clear I was *not*
going down that waterslide. EVER. I composed myself,
stood up, said *good luck* to Corinne and started down the
steps, walking past everyone in line on shaky legs. In chorus,
they started making chicken clucking noises and moving
their bent arms up and down in a *chicken-like* fashion.

The final 'straw' was when I was pointed in the direction of
the restaurant across from the bottom stair. On the menu
was the Summit Plummet Chicken Dinner. And while I had
a déjà vu like moment back to the failed Girl's Club diving
attempt, I promised myself that I would never dive again.

· liar, liar ·

In *Why I Hated Pink,* I boldly declared that I was not afraid of anything. I lied to all of you and feel the need to apologize right here, right now. I am *not* afraid of some of the things you might think. Yes, I think about the chance of cancer returning someday, but it doesn't grip me with fear.

But, I *am* terrified of the Burger King guy in the television commercials of old and develop a deep pain in my chest when I think about the #$@&%! Summit Plummet water slide in Walt Disney World.

· get out ·

"get out get out wherever you are; find a new friend; jump as

high as you can; change your favorite color; dance to a ring-

tone; follow a path; kiss upside down; take a deep breath;

leave your head in the clouds; make time; put your roof down;

wear flowers in your hair; get grass stains on your knees; turn

right when you should turn left; see things from a new

perspective; it's ok, live your life."

-   AUTHOR UNKNOWN
    And Greatly Appreciated

· labels ·

Cancer patients are under considerable pressure to remain positive. We are expected to be grateful for treatment opportunities (we are), be brave 'warriors,' fight like hell (we do), never give up or complain, and 'survive.' Sometimes there is the weight of being afraid to fail, if treatments and prayers don't work, or when our bodies have simply had enough.

To me, one of the most heroic gestures is knowing when to stop treatment and save the remaining time on this earth untethered from IVs, treatment regimes, side effects and declining quality of life. Such a decision is monumental to make, especially in a culture of high technology medicine.

While I am grateful to be a *survivor*, it doesn't mean that those of us who have a bad attitude, didn't 'fight' hard enough, have a small prayer circle, or just up and quit too soon are to blame if cancer recurs.

· attitude ·

"A positive attitude may not solve all of your problems,

but it will annoy enough people to make it worth the effort."

- HERM ALBRIGHT
  Quoted in Reader's Digest, June 1995

· work ethic ·

My father, Paul, had a tremendous work ethic. In his
eulogy, I may have mentioned he had tried to instill
his work ethic in me every day but had died trying.
Dad had a tremendous sense of humor and I'd like to
think he would have appreciated the sentiment.

The truth is that I have been working since eleven years
old; delivering Sunday newspapers with my brother Joe,
to answering phones at the church rectory, scooping ice
cream (until I broke my arm), and as a student nurse,
registered nurse, and today as an educator. Over the years,
it seemed like I *always* had a better offer to do something
other than work.

After my broken arm healed that summer, my father drove
me to the mall and urged me to apply to every business
while he waited in the car. Instead of filling out applications,
I'd browse through each store for the time it would take to
complete an application, then I'd move to the next store
without once applying for a job.

One summer over thirty years ago, Brian and I hoped to go
to the beach, but I was scheduled to work at the hospital.
We (mostly me) hatched a plan that my mother would drop
me off at work with my white uniform on. I waved goodbye
to her and walked into the lobby, with a bathing suit
underneath my uniform. After a quick change in the
bathroom at work, I was beach ready. As my mother
drove away, Brian's car pulled up and off we went to the
beach.

· worker bee ·

When I did make it to work, I think it deserves a mention that I worked hard. As the years passed, I found a lot of satisfaction in working as a nurse, often pursuing post diploma education, while raising a lively and growing family simultaneously.

After being diagnosed with breast cancer, my work self and sense of purpose were shattered, because I was unable to work for eight months. And while I realized the thrill of a 'job well done' long before this, my father's words reverberated in my bald head and I *finally* understood what he was trying to tell me. I will *never* take the opportunity to work a full day lightly again.

· fear naught ·

To My Father

A giant pine, magnificent and old

Stood staunch against the sky and all around

Shed beauty, grace and power.

Within its fold birds safely reared their young.

The velvet ground beneath was gentle,

and the cooling shade gave cheer to passersby.

Its towering arms a landmark stood, erect and unafraid,

As if to say, "Fear naught from life's alarms."

It fell one day.

Where it had dauntless stood was loneliness and void.

But men who passed paid tribute – and said,

"To know this life was good,

It left its' mark on me. Its work stands fast".

And so it lives. Such life no bonds can hold –

This giant pine, magnificent and old.

- GEORGIA HARKNESS
Copyright 1945 Abington Press.

Travis, a gifted woodworker, made a beautiful sign that hangs in our kitchen with the words, "Fear naught from life's alarms" carefully carved. It is one of my most revered gifts.

· poetry in motion ·

As like music, poetry is something to which I am naturally drawn. I not only read poetry but take a shot at writing it as well. I didn't seek poetry out, although I have been fascinated by words for as long as I can remember. I recently found a notebook from high school filled with poems I had written but forgotten about.

I am reminded of Neil Diamond's *Play Me* lyrics that include the line "rhymes that sprang from me." For the past few years, I have been unable to keep up with ideas for poems, letters, and lousy haiku. I jot down phrases and rhymes and everything I can remember that pop into my head; later piecing the words together, trying to make sense of it all.

I also do a fair amount of writing for work (manuscripts, grants, research proposals) and thoroughly enjoy it, despite its rigor. I have always said that if I could spend my days reading, writing, and running, I would be perfectly content. But I need to add poetry, photography, and my elusive quest to play the piano to that list.

· a poem comes to life ·

Mackenzie's sixth grade poem mentioned my desire to visit New York City, California, and Ireland. I am happy to report that NYC and California have since been crossed off my list, and I just returned from a conference in Ireland.

NYC was just as I had imagined and more. I went the first time with my NSBs and had a memorable trip. I have been several times since and each time, I find something new, while walking the streets exploring.

On one trip with colleagues and students, we hailed a cab to the National September 11 Memorial Museum. The driver was originally from Haiti. During the ride, we spoke about Haiti, and somehow happened on the topic of breast cancer, which she had endured.

The next time in NYC, my NSBs and I hailed a cab to a concert. And guess who the cab driver was? Yup, the same woman from the last trip. She was describing that when it was as hot and humid as that day was, the cockroaches take flight. Thankfully, we never saw anything that resembled a flying cockroach, but what are the odds of hopping in the same cab twice in NYC?

I have since traveled to Portugal, Spain, and Scotland, but now I'm getting ahead of myself.

· i had a dream ·

The fifth of eight chemotherapy rounds was one for the books. The Taxol infusion itself went well but I later had a toxic reaction that manifested itself as a fever, soaking sweats, and alarming pain in my breast. I felt like I was dying, and likely would not wake up in the morning. I tried to get comfortable and calm down; hoping to sleep for a spell.

Maybe it was the fever, or medication for pain, or perhaps I wasn't fully asleep, but I had the most overwhelming feeling of tranquility come over me. I remember thinking to myself, "That's it? This is all there is to dying?" I believe I had captured a glimpse of the other side and willed myself to remember every minute detail when I fully woke. But when I wakened, I could only recall being in a black and white silent movie with a grey 'wall' and on the other side was peace.

· hall of famer·

Twenty something years out of high school, I received a
call from my alma mater. I had been nominated for induction
into its Hall of Fame. Truth be told, when the caller identified
themselves, I thought maybe I didn't officially graduate due
to missed homework assignments or skipped detentions.

As the shyness of youth wore off, I became a bit of a rebel
and was proud of it. I was bored and restless; a perpetual
day dreamer. And through it all, I liked school if challenged,
and maintained respectable grades without doing an overabundance of work.

I was honored to be recognized for research and service-work
with underserved women; and women with breast cancer in
the community. My former biology teacher, and then Principal
Mrs. R introduced me at the ceremony and described me as
always passing in completed homework. I don't recall doing
lots of work in school, but Mrs. R failed to mention I was
expected to give a speech after her introduction.

While in the company of impressive alumni and family,
I became distracted (somethings never change) in writing
the needed speech on my phone's 'notes' app. I gave the
brief talk and before leaving for the night, snuck to see
my old locker and being back there felt like going home.

· genetic testing ·

When first diagnosed, I was on the cusp of whether I should have genetic testing because of my age. As my sisters and daughter had their annual health checkups, they were asked about my genetic predisposition. They (except for Kenzie) were fastidious in getting mammograms, but each had results requiring follow up screening.

At the next oncology appointment, we discussed the possibility of genetic testing and I was referred for screening. As the date with the genetic counselor neared, I became short-tempered. I couldn't help thinking what a mutation would mean to my family (males *and* females) and how many phone calls I would have to make to my large extended family (just kidding) if I carried the genes.

The counselor was a young woman who did a thorough history. She never once looked up while asking questions or drawing the genome map. She walked me to the lab for a blood draw. I was still feeling irritable, that quickly turned to anger when she said to the laboratory technician, "I'm sorry to ruin your day, but here's another one." The technician was lovely and skilled and tried to make up for the lack of professionalism from the counselor, but I remained angry.

The BRCA1 and BRCA2 gene results were negative and we all breathed a collective sigh of relief. As genetic testing has advanced over the past few years, I am going to have additional testing later this year.

· joy ·

"This is the true joy in life, the being used for a

purpose recognized by yourself as a mighty one;

the being thoroughly worn out before you are thrown

on the scrap heap; the being a force of Nature

instead of a feverish selfish little clod of ailments and

grievances complaining that the world will not devote itself

to making you happy."

-   GEORGE BERNARD SHAW
    Now in the public domain

· lady bug ·

When you put your heart and thoughts on paper and lob it out there, you are never certain what the reaction of the world will be. For me, the response has been overwhelmingly positive, and countless people reached out a hand. I *think* because cancer is a universal phenomenon, stories such as this resonate with people.

While in my office at work, I heard the softest knock on my door. A gentleman stood there and asked if I had time to talk. 'Of course,' I said, as meeting with and talking to people are two of my favorite pastimes. He had come across my book at a bookstore and realized we worked at the same university. He spoke of his wife, a cancer patient, who had a ladybug tattooed on her leg for each year of remission. He was proud to announce she was going for another tattoo in the weeks to come.

And while I have considered a tattoo along the way, I have three on my chest that aligned with the radiation machine during treatment. *If* I were to get a tattoo, it would simply be *Proverbs 31:25-29.* And while not a religious person, this verse has always moved me: *"She is clothed in strength and dignity, and she laughs without fear of the future. When she speaks, her words are wise, and she gives instructions with kindness. She carefully watches everything in her household and suffers nothing from laziness. Her children stand and bless her. Her husband praises her."*

· tired ·

"During chemo, you're more tired than you've ever been.

It's like a cloud passing over the sun, and suddenly you're

out. You don't know how you'll answer the door when

your groceries are delivered. But you also find that you're

stronger than you've ever been. You're clear. Your

mortality is at optimal distance, not up so close that it

obscures everything else, but close enough to give you

depth perception. Previously, it has taken you weeks,

months, or years to discover the meaning of an

experience. Now it's instantaneous."

- MELISSA BANK
  Excerpt(s) from THE GIRLS' GUIDE TO HUNTING AND
  FISHING by Melissa Bank, copyright © 1999 by Melissa
  Bank. Used by permission of Viking Books, an imprint of
  Penguin Publishing Group, a division of Penguin Random
  House LLC. All rights reserved.

· vitamins ·

At one point, my Vitamin D level was below normal. A simple blood test confirmed this, and I was encouraged to take a daily dose. Adequate levels of this vitamin may protect from certain forms of cancer, lower the risk of depression and cardiac disease, and safeguard one's immune system.

'D' has also been dubbed the 'sunshine vitamin' because skin produces it in response to sunlight and aids in its absorption. My solution to increasing the levels in my body was to move to a tropical island and bask daily in the sun. Brian was not on board with this idea (not sure why) so I continue to take a daily dose of sunshine every morning and dream of the sea.

· voice ·

My Nana was incredible to us. Since she never drove, she took the bus back and forth to work and took us kids school shopping or out for lunch. We often slept over her house, especially after my grandfather passed, and every visit was a grand adventure. The only downside to visiting was that she had two enormous oak trees in her yard and we'd rake up the fallen leaves into bags (sometimes sixty of them) with her and my dad every fall. Nana never wore pants (or sensible shoes) and joined us raking her small yard with her kitten heels on, an old coat from the back porch over her dress with an older version *multi-colored upside-down bird nest* hat atop her head.

Being the middle one of five, I often caved into what the majority wanted (until I was a teen). My grandmother was preparing lunch for us and gave us two options to choose from. I said it didn't matter to me. She replied that she wanted to know what *I* wanted, and I truly didn't care but she was waiting for a response, so I said one of the choices.

She later pulled me aside and gently whispered that I should never be afraid to ask for what I wanted or to speak my mind. To me, it didn't matter what I had for lunch, but I have taken her advice with me; she helped me find my voice that day.

· whisper ·

My beautiful, but very quiet mother, took all this breast cancer stuff hard. She is quirky and I sometimes (oftentimes) wonder where I came from. Once, when Brian, me and the kids were staying at her house for several months as our new house was being built, she called to say she was bringing ice cream home for all of us. It was summer time, and we had a lot of the kids' things in storage, so entertaining them was challenging.

A few minutes went by and I heard a car horn honking. I went outside, only to see her driving her car into the driveway. She was laughing while holding six ice cream cones that were dripping down her hands and over the steering wheel. I helped her out of the car and whispered, "Wouldn't buying a half gallon of ice cream been a better idea?" under my breath. I don't think she heard me. Then we all started to laugh and eat what was salvageable.

During treatment, I received a card from Mom with a lovely greeting and handwritten note that said, "If you need anything, just whisper." I heard *her* loud and clear and listen more closely to the whispers of those around me.

· cupcake ·

In kindergarten, the teacher celebrated each of our birthdays by bringing in a pink *Snowball* cake for the birthday boy/girl. I always thought Mrs. B was fabulous (she wore her hair in a chignon and a bright scarf tied around her neck), but this grand birthday gesture elevated her to sainthood in my eyes.

My birthday typically falls on Thanksgiving holiday break, and I began to ask my mother in early October if I would be in school on my birthday. My birthday was the day after Thanksgiving that year; therefore, this girl would *not* be celebrating her fifth birthday at school with a pink *Snowball* cake.

I was *devastated*. But quickly turned it around and felt as though I should advocate for myself and on behalf of all future kindergarteners who were denied a perfect pink cake. I asked Mrs. B if she might *consider* bringing in a cake for a student if their birthday fell on a holiday or weekend after we returned to school. She said, "Well that wouldn't be fair to the students who have summer birthdays." I realized that I may have been shy, but I was going to stick up for my rights, even though I became a little jaded that day.

I recently found *Snowball* cakes in the store, only to find they are sold in a package of two; looking like a pair of 'boobs.' Is nothing sacred anymore?

· grammie ·

My maternal grandparents raised eight children, had twenty-nine grandchildren, and over fifty great-grandchildren. Their legacy continues as there are now great, great-grandchildren.

Grammie sent greeting cards to me while I was allegedly studying in nursing school. One of my favorite things was to find a card in mailbox #63 from her. She always wrote a brief note with a five-dollar bill in the card. And always signed off with, "Don't take any wooden nickels, Love, Grammie." Thankfully, I never had the opportunity to decline a wooden nickel, but I was well-prepared in case.

In addition to not driving or wearing pants, my grandmother never drank alcohol. I hope she didn't mind that I always spent her money on beer. However, she'd likely be less impressed that my nickname in high school was Sister Mary Six Pack and it had *nothing* to do with my abs.

· on shopping ·

Grammie also shared timeless advice regarding shopping.
She had lived through The Great Depression as a young
woman and had a large family. In the rare instance she
bought a dress for herself, she would immediately hang it
in the back of her closet and not wear it for a while.

When she did finally put it on, my grandfather would
invariably ask if the dress was 'new.' As she didn't want to
lie she would honestly reply, "This ole thing? It's been in
my closet for a long time." Brilliant. Perfectly brilliant.
And this method of shopping and dodging continues to
be passed down from generation to generation.

· facebook ·

As I completed my first book, I decided to join Facebook.
I was hesitant as, like most things, there are pros and cons to
weigh out. It has been nice to have a connection to friends
from kindergarten on, relatives I may not see regularly, and
look at the world from a different perspective. One favorite
part of Facebook is that I am in contact with many of my dad's
cousins. The other is having a page dedicated to *Why I Hated
Pink*.

Once my hair started to grow back, I took my wig (the
raccoon) off for the last time, placed it back on the
Styrofoam mold stuck the wig pin in the forehead of the
mold, and ceremoniously threw it on the top shelf of my
bathroom closet as far and hard as I could. My health
insurance covered the cost of the wig ($500) and I could
get a new one in five years if needed.

Several years later, Dad's cousin asked via Facebook if I was
willing to share my wig with her dear friend. She was going
to a wedding and thought having a wig to wear would be
nice. I climbed up to reach the wig, pulled it down, washed
and styled it and met Dee for lunch with the goods in tow.
Part of me thought it might be bad karma to give the wig
away but decided this was the best possible use for it. Word
has it that her friend danced the night away. I couldn't think
of a better send off for the 'raccoon.'

· team ·

I have been fortunate in that I have had the same team of doctors for the past twelve years. There has been a change in NPs as they have moved to different positions, each providing me with wonderful care. My oncologist often calls me 'dear heart' and is bright and kind. My surgeon is matter of fact in her approach but always takes time to listen and support me. The radiologist was phenomenal, but thankfully, our time together was fleeting.

Some fellow cancer patients lament their medical teams and switch to find new ones (often more than once) who align with their philosophical, religious and health needs. I have been lucky in that there has been continuity in my care.

My primary care doctor (and his nurse) have been extraordinary to me, knowing my personality and likelihood of staying away from the office unless I was truly sick. From the start, he told me I was his favorite patient, but truth be told, he likely says that to all his patients. I have known him since he was an intern as my nursing career was beginning at a local hospital. He has saved me repeatedly, with big and little gestures and his reassuring ways.

Next spring, he will be retiring, leaving a void and a sense of uncertainty. His retirement is well-deserved, and I am on solid ground and know I can face whatever comes my way.

He has been patiently waiting for this 'sequel' to *Why I Hated Pink* for almost a decade. The very least I can do is bring along a copy of this to him in October, twelve years from diagnosis.

· motto ·

During treatment, I followed the self-proclaimed motto
'Smile anyway.' It really helped me when I smiled through
the darkness of cancer which lightened the mood for everyone
around me. Brian's idea to make t-shirts with this motto never
materialized, which is good news. When someone asks me
how I am, I reply, *'Happy, tired and blessed.'* Because I am all
those things, all at once, every single day.

· customer service ·

Typically, making a follow up appointment is an easy process, as it should be. But sometimes, it's hard to match your schedule with the provider's availability. On more than one occasion over the years, there is a back and forth of options, until finally agreeing on a date.

During one exchange, the scheduler and I were having difficulty reaching a date. I was back to work and had a full schedule. At one point I mentioned that I was *busy* again. I meant it like it was a badge of pride for me to be back in the swing, but she curtly replied, "We're all busy."

No doubt it is a daunting task fitting everyone in a tight schedule while making them happy, but there is no need to be abrupt. After all, I was busy again!

· the good patient ·

Sometimes I think I am hypersensitive to people's verbal and non-verbal cues and can sense their thoughts. Along this cancer path and its trajectory, there is a sense of impatience or dread if a patient asks too many questions about a treatment, test, or duration of a side effect or symptom.

Patients have learned to write down their concerns or questions on paper or bring along someone who can listen in for them, take notes, and anticipate questions. Understanding the health care system is complex, providers are overbooked, and their patient panel is often quite ill. The cues I received at different points in time have prevented me from reporting something new that was going on or asking questions about lingering issues.

Throughout my thirty-two years as a nurse, I have seen and heard professionals label patients as 'difficult' because of asking lots of questions. Being a *good* patient is important as to not rock the boat because we desperately need our providers attention and care. There can be an imbalance of power that prohibits us from getting answers to all our questions in a way we can understand to move forward. We must change the dialogue, so consumers of health care have the tools they need, and every question answered to maintain or improve their health.

· kristina ·

Over a year ago I was scrolling through Facebook and a post stopped me in my tracks. One of my former students had been diagnosed with breast cancer in her late twenties. And while it seems like reaching out immediately would be a gut instinct, I had to pause to be sure I wasn't dreaming. My heart broke for her; uncertainty reared its ugly head, and I finally reached out.

As Kristina wrote beautiful, honest, and poignant posts about her diagnosis, fertility treatment to harvest her eggs, eighteen months of chemotherapy, radiation, fears, and triumphs; her constant message was of the importance of parents, family, friends, hope, diet, exercise, meditation and decreasing stress. As I knew her to be as a student, Kristina remains gracious, grateful, and wise beyond her years.

Kristina, after many months of treatment, relocated to a new city to pursue the nursing job of her dreams. More recently, she completed a second surgery and twelfth intravenous infusion of chemotherapy. With 5-10 years of medication for ovarian suppression ahead, her amazing perspective on life continues to amaze and inspire me. It is an honor to know her.

· purpose ·

What if I never find what it is I am looking for as the purpose for my life? What if I find it and don't have the heart, health, or time to see it through? Or even worse, what if it completely passes me by unaware?

-   MARYELLEN

~~~~~~

"I worry
Constantly
Will the bills be paid
And the to-dos done
Will the work be finished?
Most importantly
Will I have laughed enough
And strolled to the line of the shore
Left footprints to be washed away
Met gazes with eye contact
And held enough hands?
Will I find the edges of my life
Before they close in on me?
Will I have stretched myself
To a point of purpose
That I feel finished,
    When I am done?"

-   **DR. MAYA KUCZMA**
    Permission to publish the excerpt has been requested

· martin ·

My nephew Martin was born in the hospital across town, just as I was finishing my eighth and final chemotherapy treatment eleven years ago. Today, he is a thriving middle schooler who is bright and funny and an incredible baseball player and brother. I am not sure if he knows we share a special day, as I made my way across town with Francie to meet him and visit my sister Erin and her husband.
It was quite a day and I have never forgotten his birthdate.

· pre-existing ·

At the start of 2014, health insurance companies in the U.S. could not refuse to cover or charge more for people with a pre-existing condition, or health problem before the start of new health care coverage. This was an encouraging change, especially for the one out of two Americans who have a health condition that qualifies as 'pre-existing.' I relished this victory for us all.

More recently, this law has become under fire, causing angst (and more uncertainty) as insurance companies can deny coverage for those pre-existing conditions, which seems rather unfair. Cancer, like other chronic illnesses, are a mind game. While some diseases may be preventable, many have a genetic predisposition; with cancer sometimes called a 'mistake of nature.' It seems unfair to deny care to people of all ages because they have one of many illnesses, from acne to diabetes to cancer.

· life ·

"Nobody teaches life anything."

- GABRIEL GARCIA MÁRQUEZ
  Now in the public domain

· mustang beatrice ·

One of Brian's grandmothers was like mine in that she never wore anything but dresses, and never drove a car. In stark contrast, his maternal grandmother wore jeans, drove a black Ford Mustang and enjoyed an occasional scotch and water that was never *quite* strong enough. And while I loved both, I learned that you could write your own story. It is not written down *anywhere* that we must grow up and lose our sense of wonder regardless of what life dishes out. Ever.

· little marks of kindness ·

As I was writing this book and dreading that I might be
forgotten someday, my former student Erin posted this on
her Facebook wall. The timing was perfect. I am doing the
best I can.

∧∧

"You might think you don't matter in this world, but
because of you someone has a favourite mug to drink
their tea out of each morning that you bought them.
Someone hears a song on the radio and it reminds them
of you. Someone has read a book you recommended to
them and gotten lost in its pages.

Someone's remembered a joke you told them and smiled
to themselves on the bus. Someone's tried on a top and felt
beautiful because you complimented them on it. Someone
has a memory that makes them grin that involves you.
Someone now likes themselves that little bit more because
you made a passing comment that made them feel good.

Never think you don't have an impact,
your fingerprints can't be wiped away from the little
marks of kindness that you've left behind."

-    AUTHOR UNKNOWN
      And Greatly Appreciated

· buppa ·

Mackenzie was born in May during the same period that my
Dad was dying. It was a bittersweet time, as we welcomed a
precious new daughter, but were in the final days of having
my father on this earth. To complicate our fragile emotions,
our beloved Grammie died unexpectedly in July. She sat on
her couch one afternoon watching soap operas, with a book
on her lap and never woke up. My Dad made it to her wake
and funeral (not sure how), had a beer and galumpkis at the
luncheon following her funeral mass, then went home and
slept for twenty-four hours straight. He passed away a couple
of weeks later in early August.

I had spent so much time with my mom and siblings during
that tumultuous summer that when we tried to get back to our
former lives, we found that in addition to mourning Dad and
my grandmother, we also missed being with one another
terribly. But we had to get back to children and jobs, and face
reality. I was harshly mindful that the world was still spinning
and not going to pause to pay homage to our shattered hearts.
Travis was heading to kindergarten at the end of August, so
we were getting him set to start school. I would have preferred
keeping him home forever.

My father-in-law (called 'Buppa' by Travis) was retiring in
early September. We were invited to attend a reception for the
retirees from his company and while I was thrilled for him, I
understood that my dad would not reach the milestone of
retirement. I envied the men and women being celebrated that
day for a 'job well done.' It was another stark reminder of
what he and my family had lost.

While at the reception, a man said something sexist to me and
Buppa overheard him. Buppa showed him his fist (a first for

me) and asked the man if he had "ever seen this (fist) get angry." And while it wasn't funny, we laugh about it still. He told Brian that I was a tough *cookie* and that endeared him to me forever. But more importantly, I felt safe knowing he had my back as my whole being was missing my father.

· stockings ·

As kids, my mother made each of us a Christmas stocking
that was carefully tacked to the fireplace hearth in early
December for many years. We were not able to open our
Christmas gifts before our parents woke for the day, but
stockings were fair game.

Each stocking was comprised of crocheted ivory squares,
stitched together carefully with a different color yarn.
My stocking was held together with hot pink yarn.

The December after Dad passed, we hosted Christmas Eve
in our home in Connecticut. For the weeks leading up to that
Christmas, it was common to find the tree had fallen on the
floor during the night. Brian repeatedly fixed the stand it was
in, and still, a *SWISH* sound woke us up each night. We think
Dad may have had something to do with it. He *was* always
up to something. It was the only time in our thirty years of
marriage that we had a Christmas tree that fell over.
And over again.

· pink ·

Pink and I have a sordid past. As a young girl, and into my late thirties, pink was my favorite color. I was enthralled by hot pink, like the velvet in the jewelry box my Dad made for me one Christmas, a long strand of yarn holding my childhood Christmas stocking together, and the high-top Chuck Taylor's I wore in my twenties. But the idea of missed pink *Snowball* cakes in kindergarten and the association of the pink ribbon to breast cancer left a bitter taste that is still difficult to reconcile. There was also a jump rope song that began 'Ink, pink, you stink' that I used to get in trouble for singing. You will have to look up the rest of it because it's not very nice and I was very fresh.

Recently, I came across an article by Jason Daley about bright pink color. According to smithsoniummag.org, bright pink pigments were found in fossils drilled in West Africa, making it the oldest organic color found to date. So now it's hard to 'hate' a "bit of bright pink that has survived in 1.1 billion-year-old rocks." This pigment is 600 million years older than any previous sample found.

This is a tough one. Pink is resilient, and yet I can't help but wonder if Tyrannosaurus Rex was bright pink? I may have to reconsider this pink thing. Again.

· waiting rooms ·

One complaint I have regarding waiting rooms is that I have
yet to sit in one with a stack of magazines that doesn't focus
on cancer. A distraction from cancer would be welcomed
while waiting in trepidation for an oncology appointment.
Sometimes I bring a book and get to read anywhere between
one page to one hundred pages before being called into the
examination room. Other times, I watch whatever game show
or news station is wailing on television with the highest
volume imaginable.

But at one visit, as I found a seat in the busy waiting room
hoping for a lighthearted magazine to occupy my time, I
noticed copies of *Why I Hated Pink* on the tables. One woman
was reading a copy and smiling as she turned each page.
I was frozen in my chair trying to figure out how to gauge
her reaction without being conspicuous. Thankfully, I was
called ahead of her, but my heart felt light and I hope she
enjoyed reading my words as much as I delighted in watching
her expressions.

· lisa ·

It is common for friends and acquaintances to reach out to
me if they know someone recently diagnosed with cancer.
I give my phone number to them to share with their loved
one. I am not sure how many 'pinkies' I have spoken to over
the past dozen years, but it is very humbling to have a
stranger reach out to chat. It can be very difficult to express
one's fear and concerns to their partner, children, extended
family, and friends. It's hard to not be upbeat for everyone
else since you (and the damn cancer) are the reason for
everyone's stress and worry.

 Less often, one of the doctors or nurses who took care of
me would ask if a woman or man recently diagnosed with
breast cancer could speak with me. While I never give
medical advice, I do try to support them and validate
feelings of uncertainty and offer hope. I met Lisa one day
at Panera Bread after we had spoken a few times. She was
in her thirties and had a three-year-old son. She had a great
smile with huge dimples and an equally enchanting attitude
with an 'onward and upward' motto. Today she is thriving,
as is her son.

· mark ·

My phone rang one afternoon, and I didn't recognize the number. When it rang a second and third time, I realized something was wrong. My sister's friend and his wife were trying to reach me because Mark had just been diagnosed with cancer. For men, the lifetime risk of getting breast cancer is about 1 in 833, as opposed to 1 in 8 women in the U.S. who will be diagnosed with breast cancer in their lifetime (American Cancer Society).

I dropped a *Why I Hated Pink* book off at his door and we continued to talk back and forth. He introduced me to a reporter at a local television station and she came to the house to interview me, camera crew and all. It was a lighthearted interview until she asked me to read an excerpt from my book. I opened the book and started to read from the page in front of me about my nurse Beth and started to get choked up.

When they aired the interview, I was teaching a class and didn't have an opportunity to watch it. I never like to have my picture taken, but to be on video tearing up on television was just dreadful. I never did watch the video, but I guess I am human after all.

· rebecca ·

The breast cancer community is unfortunately quite large, but luckily, consists of a group of people diagnosed with breast cancer that includes family, friends, caregivers, and support agencies. Since cancer does not discriminate, we are a diverse lot in terms of gender, age, race, ethnicity, culture, socioeconomic status and access to health care and insurance. And approximately 90% of us do not have a family history of breast cancer, so are blindsided by the news.

Of all the 15+ million people living with cancer in the U.S., I had the pleasure of meeting Rebecca, her infant daughter, and her sidekick, Audrey. Rebecca was pregnant when diagnosed and received chemotherapy during her pregnancy. Both she and her daughter, named after Mount Everest, are a force. Audrey is a philanthropist who works in fundraising for pancreatic cancer, and more recently, breast cancer. Together, they created *Pink Revolution* which aligned with the hospital where I received care, to provide support for individuals and researchers.

Rebecca, I, and others would share our experiences with people in the community, most often in schools or workplaces, to emphasize the need for everyone to be screened for cancer as recommended and listen to their bodies and act if they experience a new ache, pain or unfamiliar symptom. We also paired with the *15-40 Connection* doing similar advocacy work, with the mantra that any change in status in one's body lasting more than two weeks should be checked by a healthcare provider. The groups we encountered listened carefully and asked a lot of questions. When asked if anyone in the room knew someone with cancer, every single hand was raised at each site we visited. Advocating for oneself and others is a powerful way to give back to the community and find a way to move forward.

· sticking together ·

"Snowflakes are one of nature's most fragile things,

but look what they can do when they stick together."

-    VESTA M. KELLY

· research and prevention ·

While there have been considerable advancements associated with breast cancer in its early stages, men and women diagnosed with metastatic (cancer that has spread) breast cancer have not had the benefit of robust research on their behalf. The U.S. also lags in preventing disease (primary prevention) from ever occurring in the first place.

We understand more than ever the positive impact of healthy diet, moderate alcohol intake, not smoking and limiting exposure to carcinogens. But we don't always follow these guidelines when we could potentially decrease cancer rates and other chronic diseases in scores of people. We need to slow down and take care of ourselves.

Everything in moderation, except for love and laughter. Overdose on love and laughter.

· curtain call ·

"Enjoy your life this is not a dress rehearsal."

\-   AUTHOR UNKNOWN
    And Greatly Appreciated

· azores ·

Ten weeks into my new faculty role, I was in the airport
alone, heading to the Azores, Portugal to work on a student
exchange between the two universities with nursing students
and faculty. Truth be told, I don't think a single person on
either side of the Atlantic thought it would happen during
this trip because discussions had been underway since 1986.

I wasn't alone in the airport, per se, because I was part of a
larger itinerary on a trade mission. The problem was that
I only knew the university Chancellor from afar and
wouldn't have known one other person in the group if I
tripped over them. Once or twice during the flight, I
considered that I might be making a mistake in going,
but by then I was truly on a 'mission.' I kept thinking of
my mother's words said repeatedly to me over the years,
"Just be yourself."

The flight was uneventful, and I sat next to a very nervous
woman who I later found out was in route to see her
father-in -law before he passed. She had two connecting
flights to take before she would reach him, and we hugged
before she navigated her way to the next gate.

When I landed in the Azores, I was wonderstruck by the
landscape. We toured the island, and met with the president
of the archipelago during our five days there. When it was
time for the meeting regarding the student exchange, we were
at a long conference table at the university. There were several
discussions going on at once, and suddenly the focus was
on me and an Azorean nursing professor. Helder and I
tried to throw ideas out, but it was difficult to brainstorm
in a roomful of people. We planned to meet the next
morning over coffee to sort out the feasibility of an
exchange and iron out some plans.

· possibilities ·

Magical things happen when your heart and thinking

are open to every possibility.

· motion sickness ·

As we left the coffee behind the following morning and headed out for a ride, the island was more beautiful at every turn. Unfortunately for me, I have motion sickness and wasn't sure how I might tell my new colleague that he might have to stop the car, so I could get sick. Instead, I tried rolling down the window, and at every opportunity to stop and see a view, I would gulp as much fresh air in that I could. Then back in the car praying for a calm stomach until the next rest stop.

After twenty-seven years of missed opportunities, Helder and I had a nursing student exchange planned over a cup of coffee (tea for me) and a twisting and turning drive to see the countryside.

The first exchange was sixteen months later, and we are planning our fifth exchange as I type this (still using two fingers). To date, eighty-four students and faculty have been part of the exchange working in the Azores and U.S. with vulnerable groups.

When I finally mustered up the courage to tell Helder about the near disastrous car ride a couple of years later, he mentioned he was asked to attend the original meeting at the university at the last minute. Serendipity?

· dishes ·

In my twenties, I started to collect dishes from Portugal. Imagine my surprise two decades later when in a shop in the Azores, I saw these favorite dishes on display. I am a firm believer in serendipity as many things in life do not make sense until many years later.

It drives Brian crazy, but I typically buy one special dish that I like instead of the entire set. He has come home from work a time or two to find a freshly washed set of dishes stacked in the cabinet like they'd been there forever. I have also been known to bring furniture and puppies home, and he gets used to them all, eventually.

· watch ·

As I packed for the Azores trip, I purchased a new watch.
I had not worn one for many years, as the idea of time had
become distorted during treatment. I made the decision to
don a watch because I didn't want to appear as a rude
American looking at my phone to check the time.

While my Azorean colleagues will deny this, they are not
well known for being on time. I have always been on time or
early for everything and become quite stressed if traffic or the
like prohibit me from arriving someplace as scheduled.

The essence of time, although not as distorted now, remains
a valuable commodity to this cancer patient. Alberto, a friend
and colleague, has the perfect statement that captures my
perspective of this which is simply, "Take *your* time, don't
take mine."

During one exchange, my colleague and friend Stacey and I
were walking in Ponta Delgada in search of a cheeseburger
when she stopped and asked, "Do you know what you have
here?" I hadn't given a lot of thought to the impact of the
work we were doing but saw things from a different lens.
I knew and continue to appreciate the many opportunities
I have had and the amazing people I share my life with.

· eternity ·

"Time is too slow for those who wait, too swift for

those who fear, too long for those who grieve, too short for

those who rejoice, but for those who love,

time is eternity"

- HENRY VAN DYKE
  Now in the public domain

· chemo brain ·

My experience with 'chemo brain' has been inconsistent at best. During treatment, I was in a fog, uncertain if it was from the chemotherapeutic agents or the medications to mitigate effects of treatment. I have also blamed Tamoxifen for some of the dense fog that rolls through my brain.

But as I spend time with my friends and sisters, I realize they too forget a name, place, or song with the same regularity as I do. I have found that a brisk walk or run can clear the fog, regardless of its origin. And Brian always has the right word ready if it doesn't come to me.

I have been able to complete a PhD and write scholarly papers despite the 'fog' but am challenged in learning the Portuguese language. I have become somewhat adept at reading and understanding Portuguese, but speaking has been problematic to learn. I am not sure if it is because an exchange is a busy time, with little sleep and lots of work to complete and students to keep engaged. Or, if it is treatment related.

Thankfully, my Azorean colleagues and students speak English beautifully, but I always feel impolite in not reciprocating. Yet, I have added learning Portuguese to my poetry, photography, and playing the piano to do list.

· diving ·

As plans for the first student exchange were underway,
I was challenged by Helder to 'dive' into the Atlantic
Ocean when in the Azores. Truth be told, I will do 'almost'
anything on a dare, but *diving*? *Really*? Of course, I said
"yes" but needed to know some facts. From what height
would I be diving? From what would I be diving? Into
what would I be diving? What was the water temperature
in March? What about sharks? Fish? Weeds? Lifeguards?

This banter and one-upmanship went on for months until I
asked via Skype, "Am I *diving* or *jumping*?" "Jumping!"
was the response. Well, that changed everything.

When our group arrived in the Azores, we had to follow
through with the deal. We made our way to the pesqueiro
(fishing dock). The sea temperature that day was about 60°F
or 15°C. Having grown up swimming in the chilly ocean in
New Hampshire and Maine, this was going to be a piece of
cake.

I jumped off the dock into the cold water and came to the
surface smiling. Done. Three (as in times attempting to 'dive'
in one's lifetime) is a charm. Each time I am in the Azores,
one of my favorite things to do is 'dive.'

· laundry list ·

In addition to learning Portuguese, writing poetry,
photography, and playing the piano, I need to add
driving cross country in a wonky van and hiking the
entire Appalachian Trail to the list of things I have yet
to do. Just in case you're keeping track or want to join me.

· liz ·

Our collaborative work with the students and agencies
has brought us to some amazing places. Students and
faculty participating in the exchanges have presented at
Yale University, and in Barcelona. This summer, we were
off to Ireland to present an overview of the student exchange
as part of a recognition award. With this trip, I have now
traveled to the three places I 'would like to see' as
immortalized in Mackenzie's 6th grade poem written twelve
years ago.

On the flight home from Barcelona, a layover in Lisbon
caused a new person to sit next to me. I was napping on
and off (mostly on) when she (Liz) and I struck up a
conversation. Liz was gorgeous, and I learned that she
worked at a university in Rhode Island, about thirty
minutes from my home. Between naps, we talked about
many different subjects, from being an adult student
(she was enrolled in a master's degree program) to
learning that we both had breast cancer. When the plane
landed in Boston, we promised to stay in touch. I still had
another leg of my trip to make, praying to make it to see
my Auntie Joanne before she passed.

Liz and I have chatted sporadically over the past year.
She has a wonderful perspective on living that makes
being around her lots of fun.

· auntie jo ·

In addition to collecting dishes, I must confess that I pick up wooden/metal furniture and old prints that people leave on the side of the road. The thought of something or someone being lost calls me to act. In some respects, I have been a champion for the underdog since grade school recess, and my dissertation and community work with the student exchange have solidified my resolve in doing so.

It is common for me to put discarded pieces of furniture and other items in my car trunk, upcycle them with a fresh coat of paint and find a place of prominence for them in my home. People are no different. I am not sure 'upcycle' is the best term to use, but I do not like to see people living life on the outside looking in. Sometimes people need a boost, vote of confidence, fresh start, hug, a friend. An upcycle.

When I became aware that Auntie Joanne had a stroke and was in the intensive care unit, I went to visit. She was quite ill and did not want to be in the hospital. I liken it to her being a hornet trapped in a jar. Auntie recovered slowly and returned to her apartment which was near my home. I began to stop by once a week, then twice a week and almost daily before leaving for Barcelona. While in Barcelona, I drafted a eulogy for her as she was slowly slipping away.

She was a beautiful soul, who had overcome many challenges in her life, and came to rely on herself. I learned a lot during fifteen months of visits, but mostly she echoed my mother's sentiment that to 'be yourself' in this world is the most challenging but important thing. Thankfully, I made it home in time to say goodbye.

· be ·

Be
Be you
Be fair
Be silly
Be kind
Be open
Be smart
Be brave
Be aware
Be humble
Be fearless
Be-witched
Be yourself
Be generous
Be articulate
Be wonderstruck
Be imperfect
Be present
Be curious
Be humble
Be human
Be-autiful
Be strong
Be proud
Be funny
Be sassy
Be bold
Be love
Be joy
Be you
Be

· haiti ·

After returning to campus from the Azores, I geared myself
and ten students up for a service learning experience to Haiti
that aligned with their community health clinical experience.
I met extensively with the organization we paired with,
faculty members who had traveled there, and Haitian
stakeholders. I wanted our team to be prepared for the one-
week trip to work in a clinic outside of Port-au-Prince.

The goal was to create the first well-child clinic in the area
and bring as many medical supplies as we could. A team of
twenty-four of us (including my NSB Francie and wonderful
colleague Paula) achieved the goal, bringing over 600 lbs. of
supplies and caring for over 700 individuals. There are not
words to describe the beautiful people of Haiti we had the
privilege to meet. They love their families and want the best
for their children as we all do. It was difficult to see the wide
reach that poverty and lack of public infrastructure cast over
a country and her people.

But they are a resilient lot and taught me about the art of
nursing in healing, when there was little health care access
to the local hospital. A vast portion of my heart was left
behind after meeting a twelve-week old boy, weighing just
3.06 kg (6.7 lbs.), and his valiant mother. I hope to return one
day.

· a seagull ·

As Breast Cancer Awareness month in October arrives, or I reach another milestone, I often post something on Facebook. The comments are very humbling, sometimes funny, and always appreciated. On one such post, a friend posted a picture of a seagull. Just a seagull. Of course, I considered it's meaning and had to look it up.
∧∧

"Seagulls are spiritual messengers that demonstrate that a higher communication with guides is taking place. He shows how to see above situations with a higher clarity and teaches that there are many perspectives to consider. Seagull shows a sense of friendship and community and the cooperation that is needed for the whole to operate successfully. He teaches how to ride the currents of the mental, emotional and physical worlds. Are you going with the flow or fighting it? Are you cooperating with others? Are you open to your guides? Seagull can teach you many lessons of looking, living and being. It is time to listen and watch for the nuances and timing of action.

The Seagull knows that freedom is a state of mind and of the heart. Seagull can teach you to let your heart soar on the wings of freedom and joy, no matter where you are and no matter what you are doing. Seagull will help lift you out of the sands of worry and petty concerns and into the soaring heights of being one with all that is: one with the ocean,

one with the land, one with the vast and glorious sky.
The Seagull will also teach you perspective. Whenever
you care to, Seagull will take you for a ride, up into the sky
and across the wide ocean, where you will see that your
cares are as small as the grains of sand on the beach.
Seagull will teach you that your power is limitless and
unbounded and that all you need to do is stretch out your
wings and let life carry you."

- TED ANDREWS
  Permission to publish the excerpt has been requested

∧∧

And while I do not know if this was the intent of the seagull
photo, I do know for certain I have never looked at a seagull
the same way since.

· messages ·

Dad passed away one early morning in August at the age
of fifty-five. Brian and my sister Erin were with him (my mom
was resting). I was home with the kids who were five, three
and ten weeks old. My sweet NSB Francie slept over, so she
could watch the kids if I had to leave in the middle of the
night. When Brian called that Dad had passed, Francie fell
out of bed because the ring seemed loud enough to wake
the world, and we hadn't slept a whole lot, dreading the
call.

I hopped out of bed, called my sister Karen who lived
twenty minutes away, who remarkably was at my door in
an instant. We planned to travel to my parents' house
together. As I turned on the bedroom light, the bulb burned
out, the same thing happened in the bathroom, then the light
over the kitchen sink blew out, as did the microwave light
(who knew there *was* one). Francie and I were a little freaked
out but laughing at the same time. When Karen arrived in
her car with a newly burnt-out headlight, we were laughing
and crying at the same time.

To this day, as the anniversary of my father's death nears,
my siblings and I always report that lightbulbs in our
houses burn out with a flip of the switch. Coincidence or
not, I think it is his way of letting us know he is near.

· cathy ·

After graduating from nursing school, many of my classmates worked at the same hospital. Cathy was one of them. I would often see her during a patient transfer to the nursing unit she worked on or vice versa. I hadn't seen her in several years, except at a graduation party for my nephew and on one other occasion when we found ourselves dressed alike in pink flowered hospital gowns in the mammography suite waiting room.

We spoke briefly, as I waited on the radiologist to read my films because of a new lump in my breast post treatment. I assumed she was there for a routine exam, but we never had a chance to catch up because I was called back for the results.

I later learned that Cathy had been diagnosed with colon cancer. She passed away soon after my nephew's party, leaving three children and her high school sweetheart behind. In solidarity, her family rode in the Pan Mass Challenge that summer to raise money for Dana-Farber Cancer Center resources to "discover cures for all cancers." My NSB Moke, cousin John, and friend Cindy also ride in the Pan Mass.

I will not, and will never, forget Cathy's beautiful blue eyes or her infectious laugh. And so, I press on.

· menopause ·

As my cancer was diagnosed at the age of 41, no one was quite certain if I would go through menopause because of chemotherapy or not. During chemo, the hot flashes were all-consuming and ferocious. The best way to describe myself was as being a human furnace. The fires of perimenopause continue to burn, but without as much fervor. My body has yet to give in to menopause, but my periods are now many months apart.

My dissertation work with this phenomenon was eye-opening. Not so much from a menopause perspective but because of the idea that chemotherapy-induced premature menopause was daunting to the women enrolled in the study, but not the most worrisome as they balanced that along with many other things in their lives.

There is an off-Broadway show *Menopause the Musical* that I saw with my Mom, sisters, and cousin before I was diagnosed with cancer. It was hilarious and enlightening. My only problem with it is that I haven't been invited to be part of the cast. Perhaps my lack of singing and dancing skills is more widely known than I imagined. I do think I am well suited to sing about chocolate cravings, hot flashes, memory loss, and fatigue if a spot becomes available.

· then there were six ·

When the college years were winding down, Ashley, Emily and Anthony joined our family. Travis and Ashley were married last year, and Tyler and Emily's wedding is planned for next year. Both couples have homes of their own and our home has lost its constant hum of noise. Mackenzie is back in school to become a nurse, and Anthony is a state trooper. They are all working hard and are good people, the finest people. I am proud of each of them. When they are together, there is laughter and plenty of shenanigans. It is both exhilarating and exhausting.

When Kenzie composed her sixth-grade poem, she asked me what my fears were. As I mentioned, I was afraid of who would look after her if I was gone. Of course, I knew my sisters and sisters-in-law were there for her, but she now has *two* sisters who have embraced her as their own. Together, and apart, they are a mighty force.

"Every time they smile, heaven blows in"

- AUTHOR UNKNOWN
  And Greatly Appreciated

· riding shotgun ·

I often have a long commute back and forth to work.
When the kids were little, I commuted from Connecticut to
the hospital in Massachusetts and back as I worked the 3-11
shift. My dad did not like me traveling alone late at night
and bought me one of the first 'bag' cell phones for my car.

After he passed, I could feel his presence in the car on the
ride home. He wasn't 'there' after every shift ended, but he
was a regular passenger for about six months. It made me
calm as I made my way home. I didn't ever put the radio on;
I just drove in silence.

One night, I mentioned to him in the nicest way possible
that I felt safe driving alone at that hour. While I relished his
commitment, I wanted him to know I was okay. He never
rode shotgun with me after our one-sided conversation,
but I do still feel his presence. When I do see him again,
I plan to hand him the tab for the lightbulbs we purchase
every August and October.

· numbers ·

It has been said that there are signs that let us know you are 'in alignment' with the universe if we listen to them. One of these signs are in the form of numbers. People often see repetitive numbers: 111 or 222. These are called 'angel numbers.'

For many years, if I am stressed or overtired and see the numbers 1234 or 1127 (my birthdate) on a clock, receipt, phone number or anyplace, I know that everything will be okay. As I began writing this book several years ago, the title was Five Octobers, then Six Octobers...and finally as I finished writing, *Twelve Octobers*. When penning this edition, I frequently began to see the numbers 1012 or 1210. Dad's birthday is October 12 (1012) and this book is twelve Octobers (1210) and not surprisingly, my lucky number has always been twelve since it was plastered on the back of my softball uniform.

And maybe it's a coincidence the Christmas tree kept falling over after my Dad passed, and lights burn out each year near his anniversary and birthday. But somehow, I don't believe in coincidences anymore; coincidence is the universe's way of being anonymous.

· wedding bells ·

Travis and Ashley were married on the 4th of July which
happened to land on a Tuesday. The venue was in
Vermont and we had a wonderful few days together.
They had written their own vows and the day was perfect
in every way. Being the mother of the groom, Travis and I
decided early on which song we would dance to. He couldn't
listen to it though, because this *self-proclaimed man of steel*
shed tears when it came on the radio.

We both knew the words to *Danny's Song* by heart because
I sang it (off key) when rocking him as a baby (he didn't
seem to mind). As we were called to the dance floor, I was
feeling proud and bursting with joy. He had wanted me to go
in with 'guns a blazing' to the theme song from *The Good, The
Bad and The Ugly* film. I had a completely different idea in
mind that we agreed to right before our dance began. I simply
put my hand to my side to signify that he was once a little boy,
then raised my hand to the top of his head (on my tiptoes) to
show how time passed and he was now a man.

As *Danny's Song* started, my man of steel started to cry.
I was doing my best to keep it together as we were in the
middle of a circle of family and friends but was struggling to.
I did the only thing I could think of; I started singing the
lyrics to him as I did when he was a baby. I was singing, we
both were crying (from my singing?) and the wedding guests
began to sing along with us. The words "People smile and
tell me I'm the lucky one, and we've just begun, think I'm
gonna have a son" rose to the rafters and the world paused
for a moment. There wasn't a dry eye in the place and I
realized I had been part of another life milestone and
cherished every second of it. Travis, please save a dance for
me at your brother's wedding.

· travis ·

Reflections from Travis

I'll be honest I realized I took a major moment of my life for granted when Mom asked me to write a reflection piece for this upcoming book on breast cancer. But more on that later...

The topic of breast cancer has been one that I haven't mentioned to many people. When I found out about Mom's diagnosis I never wanted support from others. I felt as though I needed to be the support structure. That it was 'my job' to help support our family, and a feeling that I shouldn't burden others with what we were dealing with.

I remember my roommate Rob sheepishly asking me during our first year in college if I ever needed anything, I'd have to ask *him*. This was the last time he would ask me; he knew my personality very well.

Tyler, Mackenzie, and I are strong willed, and I credit that directly to Mom. We never showed much emotion throughout the entire process but remained supportive. It is what Mom wanted us to do.

Now back to that overlooked moment, and 'lack' of emotion I have shown over the years. When Mom asked me to write this reflection piece, I realized that I *am* an emotional person and that became clear on my wedding day. I shed some tears when seeing my then future wife walk down the aisle but shed even more as my mother and I danced to Loggins & Messina.

I only began to smile and dry my tears when I heard Rob begin singing the lyrics to "Danny's Song." Mackenzie wasn't as lucky as I was. She sobbed for the rest of the wedding.

Poor Anthony, what a trooper (no pun intended) he was! I have reminisced about that moment many times since our wedding and get a little glassy eyed thinking back to the exact moment we met in the middle of the dance floor in the wooden barn. I never realized how important that moment was. *What if* crossed my mind when I started to write this reflection piece. *What if* the outcome of her diagnosis had been different and I didn't share this moment with my mom and hear Rob's awful rendition of "Danny's Song?" I don't mean to be grim and morbid, I only mean to elucidate that anyone reading this cannot take any moment for granted.

I may not have realized how incredible that quick moment in time was for me. How it changed me for the better; how reflecting on simple moments in life can make you better. Appreciate the little things in life, they end up meaning more than anything you may be worrying about.

I still can't read *Why I Hated Pink.* I have tried so many times. I get to a certain point in the book and that stoic, rigid Travis that some of you know starts to crack.

Thank you, Mom, for asking me to write a reflection piece. It made me realize how much more our dance meant to me than I had originally thought. Love you!

- TRAVIS M. BRISBOIS

· possibilities ·

While I love teaching and the opportunities I have had across the globe, I do think about what else might be out there for me. I have many ideas of what I might like to do, but two stand out. I have an immense interest in becoming a hospice nurse. It has been kicked around in my mind since I was a novice nurse. Taking care of Auntie Joanne fueled my interest in that nursing role. But not just yet.

The other, less serious but equally enchanting opportunity would be to open a coffee shop (I promise someone else will make the coffee) and have a farmer's market with local goods and offer breakfast, lunch, and a welcoming place with amazing Wi-Fi to work, write, read, or catch up with friends. I have found the perfect location in the old fire station in town, that is not for sale...yet. I have always wanted to be a barista and will be. But not just yet.

I have even considered teaching abroad for a semester, opening an outdoor flower stand on Grafton Street in Dublin, Ireland, scooping ice cream in Pitlochry, Scotland, selling books in Cambridge, MA or serving lobster with extra butter and napkins in Perkins Cove, Maine. The possibilities are endless, but patience and timing are required.

· more on patience ·

"Be patient with yourself while you travel the road back to health"

- LISA GILLESPIE

"Patience is the art of concealing your impatience"

- GUY KAWASAKI

And this: My favorite

"Patience is a virtue, but impatience gets things done"

- CHELSEA CLINTON

· i am ·

Who I Am Not; And So, I Am

I LOVE
to sing and dance but am not Terpsichore,
to write but am not Seshat,
justice but am not Dike,
wine but am not Dionysus,
history but am not Clio,
the spirit of hope but am not Elpis,
the psalms but am not Polyhymnia,
to run but am not Atalanta,
the moon but am not Phoebe,
writing poetry but am not Brigid,
wisdom but am not Athena,
the sea but am not Amphitrite,
to speak but am not Fabulinus,
the stars but am not Asteria,
love but am not Aphrodite,
life but am not Pachamama,
beauty but am not Venus,
sleep but am not Nyx,
owls but am not Hecate,
flowers but am not Chloris,
peace but am not Harmonia,
to swim but am not Salacia,
to laugh but am not Baubo,
good health but am not Hygea,
the earth but am not Gaea,
books but am not Baalat,
dawn but am not Eos,
to think but am not Metis,
to sew but am not Rhapso,
being a nurse but am not Aceso,

to travel but am not Abeona,
dreaming of the future but am not Antevorta,
mischief but am not Até,
the mountains rise but am not Cybele,
to see but am not Theia,
being a mom but am not Rhea,
the stars but am not Ourania,
home but am not Hestia,
rain but am not Talaya,
strength but am not Bia; and,
I love the sun but am not Medusa.

I am just me, not a deity or a goddess, but an imperfect
amalgamation of everything I love, a brown-eyed girl in
hand-me-downs (thank you Janice Ian), Jill of all trades and
mistress of few, but I am not a fool. My ancestors made
sure of that.

My family, friends, colleagues, and the scores of patients
and students I have encountered have kept me humble.
I have encountered more wins than losses and wear my
heart and brain out every day. I am happy, tired, and
blessed and hope to continue but will go when I am needed.

· truth ·

"I hope to arrive to my death late, in love and a little drunk."

- ATTICUS
  Permission to publish the quote has been requested

· unmentionables ·

There is a small funeral parlor in town that reminds me of the Munster's House at 1313 Mockingbird Lane. When I drive by, I always think Herman, Lily and Grandpa are going to be on the front porch dressed in black. Brian knows I don't like it there but jokes that is where I'm going to end up.

Instead there is a funeral parlor in Oxford, MA where no members of the Munster family have been spotted. Also, in Oxford near a police station and school, the North Cemetery abuts a ball field, where people walk and run, kids ride their bikes and teenagers drink (not confirmed, but I'm quite certain). I think the activity and noise would make me content. I would also be in good company as Clarissa Harlowe aka 'Clara Barton' Founder of the American Red Cross and 'Angel of the Battlefield' is buried there.

St. Denis Church in Douglas is a fine choice for my funeral, although you may have to fill years of empty and overdue envelopes for the collection. Another thought is St. Stephen's Church in Worcester where I was baptized and attended countless masses. The drawn-out procession from church through Auburn and into Oxford could annoy a lot of people on the roads. And the funeral mass is planned, subject to change as most things are.

I would like a nice funeral program with no typos or photos of me. Please don't forget the laminated cards later thrown in mourners' top bureau drawers after arriving home. I'd appreciate white flowers like Dad loved with bold pink flowers in the spray. And bring along some pink *Snowball* cakes *just in case* the line is long.

· funeral mass ·

Entrance Hymn
Gather Us In (M. Haugen)
Be Not Afraid (B. Dufford)

First Reading (Old Testament) Ecclesiastes 3:1-8

Responsorial Psalm Psalms 139: 9-10

Second Reading (New Testament) Corinthians 12:31-13:8a

Gospel Reading Matthew 5:1-12a

The Liturgy of the Eucharist: Preparation Song
Prayer of St. Francis/Make Me A Channel of Your Peace
(S. Temple)
Here I Am Lord (D. Schutte)

Communion Hymns
I Am the Bread of Life (S. Toolan)
You are Mine (D. Hass)

Song of Farewell
On Eagle's Wings (M. Joncas)

Recessional Hymns
How Great Thou Art (traditional)
Let There Be Peace on Earth (J. Jackson & S. Miller)

Cemetery *(Please sing loud enough so Clara Barton can hear you)*
Amazing Grace (traditional)
Let it Be (P. McCartney & J. Lennon)
Imagine (J. Lennon)
Danny Boy (F. Weatherly)

· no one cares ·

"Every fucking day gets harder and harder. This disease

is a monster, a bully, and a thief.

We are being erased one at a time and no one cares."

- SUSAN RAHN
  Permission to publish the quote has been obtained

· me ·

I do not consider myself a survivor. Well, technically
according to some hazy definition I am, but bristle at the
word. I did not survive any of the great atrocities of the world:
War, famine, hate, discrimination, hunger, genocide,
loneliness, poverty, homelessness, violence, or dictatorship.
But each day I struggle to balance levity and brevity. Levity
always wins. *Every single day.*

The numbers are staggering. In 2016, there were 15,533,220
people living with cancer in the U.S., with > 20 million
people living with cancer projected in 2026 (cancer.org).
Most of you wouldn't recognize us as such. We are either
newly diagnosed, waiting for a phone call with test results,
going through treatment, living with metastatic disease, or
deemed cancer free; all of which are equivalent to standing
in quicksand.

We work hard, play hard and love hard. I imagine we all
hope for longevity. And if you complain to us about traffic
or a parking ticket, we really don't care. *Not even a little bit.*
I can go many days and weeks without the weight of the
breast cancer diagnosis received nearly twelve years ago.
It can sometimes creep in my brain even with my innate
stubbornness, especially at follow up visits. Okay, *always* at
follow up visits.

Let's just say that not one of us knows what the future holds.
If I get news that is not what I hoped for, I have been there
before. Even with good news, it takes a couple of days to
brush myself off and get back in the ring; I have climbed over
the ropes a time or two. There is still so much left to plan and
do, geography to explore and people to connect with. And
today and every day thereafter, I am not a survivor; I am me.

The End

for now

"Lovely to see you again my friend,

Walk along with me to the next bend."

-   THE MOODY BLUES

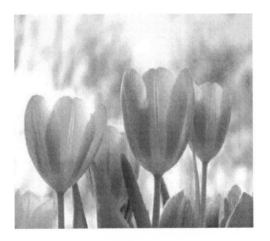

Made in the USA
Middletown, DE
12 November 2018